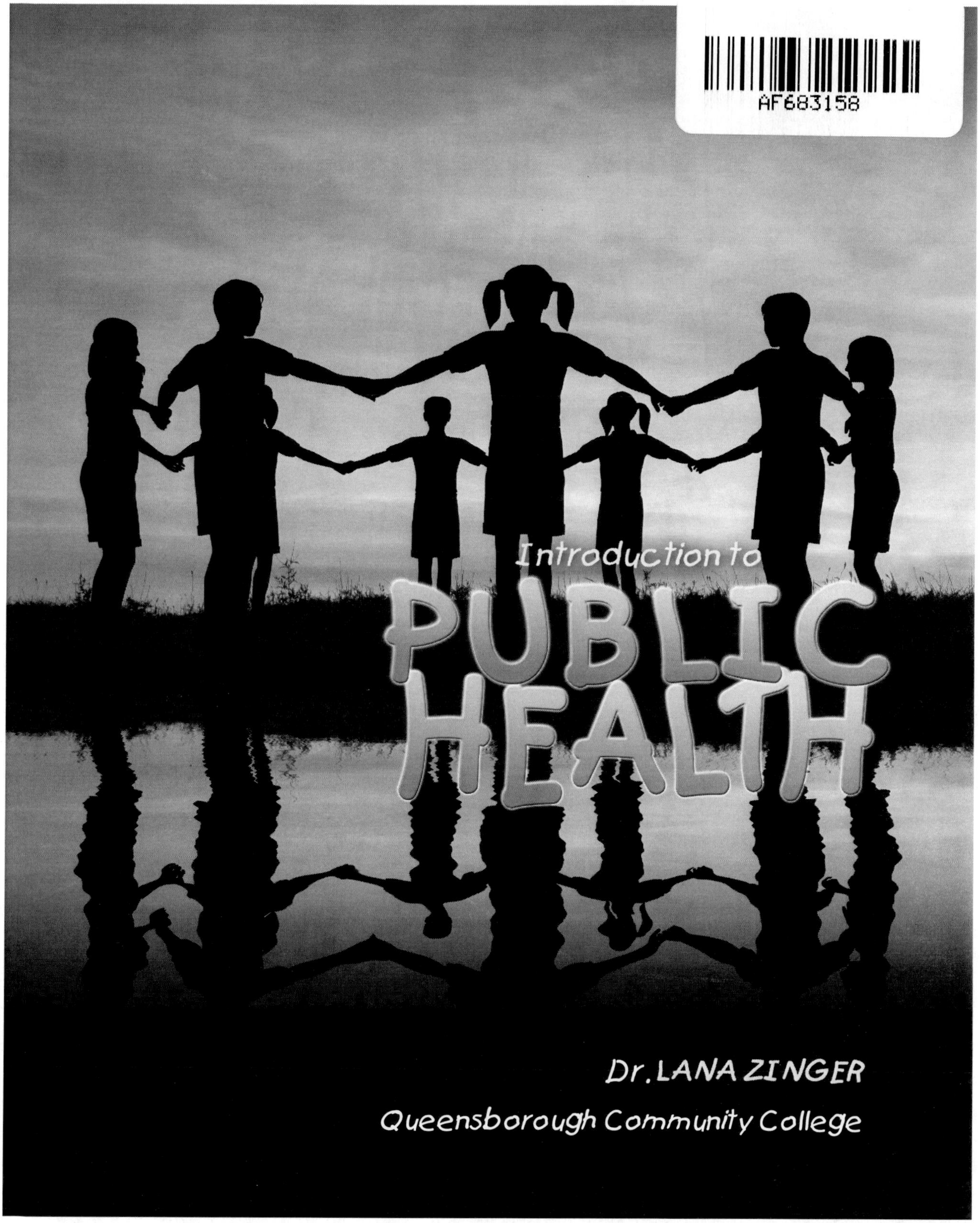

Introduction to PUBLIC HEALTH

Dr. LANA ZINGER
Queensborough Community College

Kendall Hunt
publishing company

Cover image © Shutterstock, 2010

Kendall Hunt
publishing company

www.kendallhunt.com
Send all inquiries to:
4050 Westmark Drive
Dubuque, IA 52004-1840

ISBN 978-0-7575-6830-5

Printed in the United States of America
10 9 8 7 6 5 4 3 2

Contents

1 Introduction 1
2 Creating Healthy Communities 9
3 Prevention and Control of Diseases 19
4 Health Disparities 41
5 Nutrition 55
6 Environmental Health 77
7 Health Care System 95
8 Current Issues in Global Health 105

Dedication

To my sons Max and Alexander who have greatly enriched my life with their healthy attitudes, spirited personalities, and very high energy levels. I hope the top priority in your lives will be your health, and I encourage you to enrich the communities where you live and work and always set aside time to help improve the lives of those in need.

> ***"Nation needs youthful idealism more than ever. Young people will take responsibility for making their communities stronger. They know that each of us has something to contribute. And they are ready to lead the way. There are few things more rewarding than watching young people recognize they have the power to enrich not only their own lives, but the lives of those around them as well."***
>
> **—Michelle Obama, 2009**

Chapter 1

INTRODUCTION

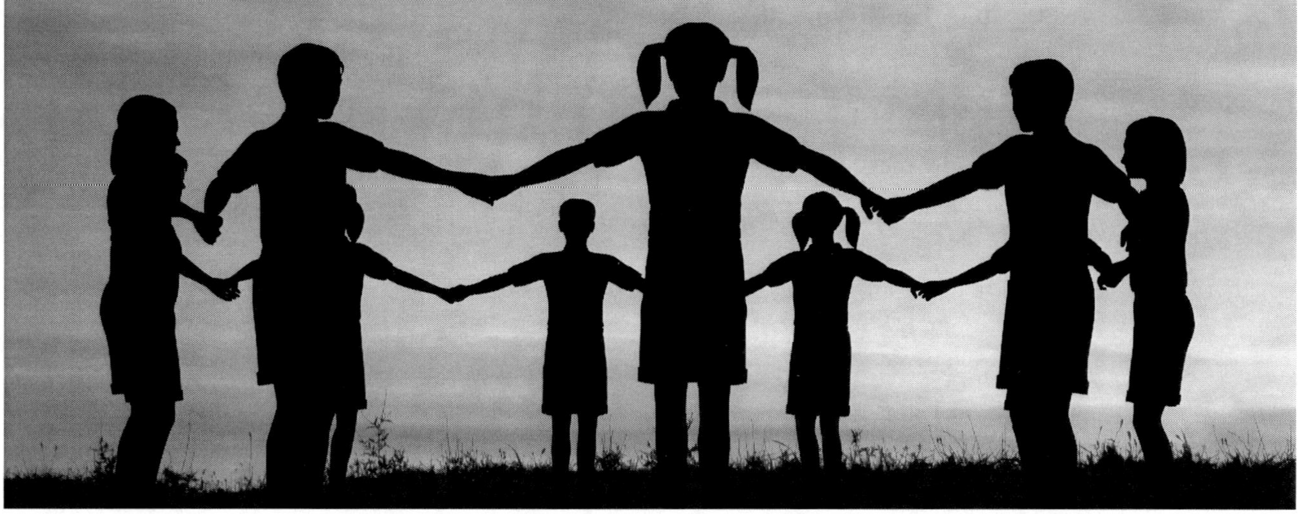

Why Should You Care About Public Health?

Health is a fundamental human right, just like water, food, and shelter. Because health is a human right, then basic health care should be available to all people. Unfortunately, millions of people around the world and in our own communities do not have access to basic levels of health care. An injustice is being committed if health care is denied because of where people are born, because of how much money they have, or as a result of other special circumstances.

Some personal health practices—such as eating well, washing hands, getting vaccinated, and practicing methods of stress reduction—can keep us healthy. However, globalization is connecting our health maintenance to the health practices of others, which is changing our health experience. For example, if immigrants arrive in our cities with untreated illnesses (tuberculosis, for example), then we are at risk for those illnesses. If our food supply comes from places where proper sanitation practices are not followed, then we are at risk for food-borne illness. To ensure that we maintain quality health care and, thus, our own health, we not only must protect our own health by the aforementioned personal health practices but also must advocate for the health of others in our own communities and globally.

The goals of this book are to increase your awareness of global health issues, to generate concern about those issues, and to help you create solutions to fix some of these issues. My hope is that you will do whatever you can to help shape a healthier world for future generations.

The World Health Organization

The World Health Organization (WHO), as a global authority within the United Nations system, is responsible for setting standards on health matters and provides global surveillance and assessment of health-related trends. In its "Preamble to the WHO Constitution," the WHO defines *health* as "[a] state of complete physical, mental and social well-being and not merely the absence of disease or infirmity" (World Health Organization, 1946). The implication is that health is not just a matter of being free of disease. Rather, it also involves nutritional and physical aspects as well as spiritual and intellectual components.

The same WHO document (WHO, 1946) expanded on the definition of *health* by laying out principles that member "States" of the United Nations were encouraged to uphold. This document emphasized that people have a fundamental right not only to health but to "the highest attainable standard of health" and that this right is not to be determined by race, religion, political belief, or economic or social condition.

The principles set forth by WHO (1946) described this high standard of health as being fundamental to "the attainment of peace and security" and indicated that it was dependent on complete cooperation—by individuals *and* "States." The WHO document put forth the belief that any state achieving "promotion and protection of health" would be of value to everyone, which affirms the premise discussed earlier that health is a global issue. Continuing in the realm of global concerns, the constitution preamble discussed the "common danger"—in regard to communicable disease, in particular—of different countries having unequal development in health promotion and disease control.

The preamble discussed the healthy development of children and how living harmoniously in a changing global environment is essential to that development. Also essential to the attainment of health is the dissemination of medical, psychological, and related knowledge to "all peoples." The principles indicate that an informed opinion and active cooperation by the public are "of the utmost importance in the improvement of the health of the people" (WHO, 1946).

Finally, WHO declared that governments have a responsibility for the health of their "peoples," a responsibility that can be achieved only by providing adequate health and social measures (WHO, 1946).

Possibly as an extension of the 1946 principles, the European World Health Organization listed specific "fundamental conditions and resources" that must be met to achieve a quality standard of health (WHO, Europe, 1986). These include peace, shelter, education, food, income, a stable ecosystem, sustainable resources, social justice, and equality.

Community Health

Before discussing global issues, we take a brief look at how health impacts—and is impacted by—communities. Continuing with the descriptions presented by WHO (1946), a *community* is a group of people with a shared location, shared environment, and shared fate. *Community health* includes both private and public efforts of individuals, groups, and organizations to promote, protect, and preserve the health of those in the community. (Note that *promote, protect,* and *preserve* are terms that were also discussed in connection with the responsibilities of "States" in the earlier discussion of principles set forth by WHO.) Neighborhoods, developments, school districts, towns, or counties make up *communities of residence.* The people that make up these communities are termed *communities of relationships*.

Global and Public Health

Global health, which is health that crosses national borders, is a huge concern because modern transportation allows infectious diseases to spread across the world at an alarming rate. Diseases are spread not only from person to person but also, as mentioned earlier, from persons to food supplies and from food supplies to persons; and the list goes on.

The developing world still suffers from largely preventable infectious diseases, mainly caused by malnutrition and poverty. Discrepancies regarding access to health care and public health initiatives between developed nations and developing nations still exist, and a large majority of disease and mortality in the developing world results from and contributes to extreme poverty.

One of the most relevant factors for increased preventable diseases globally is that many public health infrastructures are still in the process of formation throughout the world. Another concern is that not enough trained health workers or monetary resources are available to provide medical care or to work at disease prevention.

All governmental efforts to promote, protect, and preserve the people's health comprise what is termed *public health*. Threats to the overall health of a community (big or small) are considered to be a part of public health and are based on *population* health analysis. The "population" in question can be as big as a handful of people or several continents.

As can be seen, *public health* is no small entity; it encompasses other fields of health, including environmental, social, behavioral, and occupational health.

The focus of a public health intervention is to prevent rather than treat a disease, especially through the promotion of healthy behaviors. Examples of public health measures include vaccination programs and distribution of condoms.

Factors That Affect the Health of a Community

Not only physical factors but also social and cultural factors can influence the health of a community. Some *physical factors* that affect a community's health are listed here with some examples that demonstrate how these factors can impact the community.

- Geography: Parasitic diseases
- Environment: Availability of natural resources
- Community size: Overcrowding
- Industrial development: Pollution

Some *social and cultural factors* that can influence a community's health follow. These, too, are presented with examples of how these factors can impact the community.

- Beliefs, traditions, and prejudices: Availability of ethnic foods, racial disparities
- Economics: Health-care benefits
- Politics: Government participation and funding
- Religion: Beliefs about medical treatment
- Social norms: Drinking on a college campus
- Socioeconomic status (SES): Number of people below poverty level

An empowered community includes partnerships among residents, local institutions, and associations to improve community health. The quality and effectiveness of community organizing can affect the community's health by such activities as implementing taxes and after-school programs. In addition, community empowerment can be affected by what health agencies are available. Is there a local health department? Are there voluntary health agencies? If partnerships are created, the partnerships must have the ability to solve problems. That is, they must be able to organize to lobby for change at the city level, and they must be taken seriously by the city council.

Included in social and cultural factors are lifestyle choices or individual behaviors, which are major causes of mortality in the United States. A **lifestyle choice** or modifiable behavior is something that a person has some control over; that is, the person can choose whether or not to participate in the behavior. Examples include exercising, smoking (starting or stopping), and eating healthy. If an individual cannot access the information or the tools (such as healthy food or money to obtain healthy food), then the "choice" becomes a community issue.

Modern Public Health

As the rate of infectious diseases in the developed world decreased throughout the 20th century, public health began to put more focus on chronic diseases such as heart disease. In the United States, most adults die from chronic illnesses rather than from infectious diseases. (Accidents are the leading threat to children in the United States.)

During the 20th century, the health and life expectancy of persons residing in the United States improved dramatically. During this period, it was recognized that the greatest potential for improving the health of communities and populations was not through health care but through health-promotion and disease-prevention programs.

Public Health Achievements in the United States in the 20th Century

Some of the programs that contributed to the dramatic improvement in health and life expectancy in the United States during the 20th century are discussed in this and subsequent paragraphs (Centers for Disease Control and Prevention, 1999). One of the most cost-effective tools for prevention of disease, disability, and even death is *vaccination*. The United States experienced success in the 20th century by using vaccines to eradicate smallpox; eliminate polio; and control measles, rubella, and tetanus. Other public health programs implemented to *control infectious diseases* included a focus on clean water and improved sanitation. Control of tuberculosis and sexually transmitted diseases (STDs) was greatly enhanced by the discovery of *antimicrobial therapy.*

An emphasis on *motor-vehicle safety* led to safer vehicles and increased use of safety features such as seat belts, child safety seats, and motorcycle helmets. Also included in this category were stricter laws and enforcement regarding drinking and driving. All of these changes have resulted in reductions in motor-vehicle-related deaths.

In the early 21st century, we have experienced some highly publicized accounts of mining and workplace-related injuries and deaths. However, changes made during the 20th century with the intent of having *safer workplaces* actually led to decreases in severe injuries and deaths related to mining, manufacturing, construction, and transportation.

Another focus of 20th-century health-promotion programs was "food-fortification programs," which were designed with the intent of creating *safer and healthier foods*. These programs have led to the near elimination in the United States of *nutritional-deficiency diseases* such as rickets, goiter, and pellagra. Nutrition also played a role in programs designed especially for *healthier mothers and babies*. Not only nutrition but also better prenatal care and technological advances in maternal and neonatal care led to decreases in infant and maternal mortality.

Another area credited with having decreased the number of infant, child, and maternal deaths was *family planning*, in particular, *access* to services. Provision of contraceptive services and access to sexual health education were instrumental parts of the family-planning programs implemented in the 20th century in the United States.

It was during the 20th century that *tobacco use as a health hazard* was recognized. Students who watch some of the television reruns from the 1950s, 1960s, and 1970s may be surprised at the amount of cigarette and cigar smoking that was considered acceptable—and even a sign of affluence—during that time. The 20th century saw the beginning of smoking-cessation programs and smoke-free zones and the beginning of the end of television advertisements, which all contributed to the reduction of smoking-related deaths.

Life Expectancy

Life expectancy in the United States continues to improve. The average life expectancy for Americans is 77.6 years, a record high according to the latest statistics from the Centers for Disease Control and Prevention (CDC). However, people in the United States still have a somewhat lower life expectancy than those of other developed countries. Because many infectious diseases are controlled and Americans are living longer, it is not surprising that chronic health problems, which are often associated with aging (e.g., heart disease, cancer, stroke, and lung disease), are among the leading causes of illness and death. Some conditions are wholly or partly the result of individual choices about smoking, diet, or exercise; but other health problems may be associated with exposure to environmental pollutants.

Some selected life expectancies follow:

- White males: 75.4 years
- Black males: 69.2 years
- White females: 80.5 years
- Black females: 76.1 years

Though accidents are the leading cause of death for those under age 34 years, in older age groups, chronic diseases are the leading causes. In fact, as shown in the accompanying box, the top two causes of death for males and females in the United States in 2000 were heart disease and cancer (Mokdad, Marks, Stroup, et al., 2004).

Top Ten Leading Causes of Death for Americans

1. Heart disease
2. Malignant neoplasms
3. Cerebrovascular diseases
4. Chronic lower respiratory diseases
5. Accidents
6. Diabetes mellitus
7. Influenza and pneumonia
8. Alzheimer's disease
9. Nephritis, nephrotic syndrome, nephrosis
10. Septicemia

Well over a third of all deaths in the United States could be attributed to a limited number of largely preventable behaviors and exposures including smoking, poor diet and physical inactivity, and alcohol consumption. Changing these modifiable behaviors can increase a person's life expectancy or longevity and prevent early death.

Top Three Leading Causes of Preventable Death in the United States

1. Tobacco use (smoking)
2. Poor diet and physical inactivity
3. Alcohol consumption

Better Health in the 21st Century

Currently, there is a global health crisis, characterized by growing inequalities within and between countries. Globalization has led to the inequitable distribution of resources necessary for people's health, particularly that of poor people. For example, millions of poor, landless farmers have lost their livelihoods; millions of people in poor countries urgently need HIV treatment, yet less than 5% have access to the needed drugs; and millions of people have lost health insurance.

Current public health challenges are many and exist not only in the United States but also globally—and probably to a greater extent in countries experiencing the inequities already mentioned. First among the challenges are *health-care delivery and access to care*. In the United States, the number of people without health insurance has continued to grow, a situation that impedes our nation's health and productivity. Included in these challenges are the *inequalities* or *health disparities* that exist between different ethnic or racial groups and for those in low socioeconomic positions.

Even with advances made in the areas of smoking-cessation programs, as previously mentioned, the fact remains that *smoking is deadly and addictive.* It accounts for nearly one in five deaths in the United States. Critics believe that tobacco companies put greed and profit above health, ethics, and decency and continue to modify their products to make them even more addictive and attractive.

A very serious challenge is the need to *focus on safe, healthy, and affordable food.* Every 2 hours, one person in the United States dies from contaminated food. This challenge includes the task of ensuring that nutritional needs are being met.

Environmental pollution is an ongoing challenge and includes the risk to individuals and to the planet. The rise of pollution is blamed for climate changes and changes to our food supply. Pollution also increases the risk of diseases, not the least of which is asthma.

Lifestyle diseases remain as some of the leading killers of people in the United States. Obesity and its associated problems (i.e., diabetes and cardiovascular) are largely preventable in most people. Education is needed to assist people in making personal choices that enable them to obtain optimal health.

Problems also continuing to affect our communities are *alcohol and drug abuse* and *untreated mental disorders.* As can be seen, these challenges and others will guide the efforts of educators and people who are looking toward the future with a sense of responsibility regarding what can and must be achieved in the years to come.

References

Anonymous. (1997). The sixth report of the Joint National Committee on Prevention, Detection, Evaluation, and Treatment of High Blood Pressure. *Archives of Internal Medicine, 157*, 2413–2446.

Bolen, J. R., Sleet, D. A., Chorba, T., et al. (1997). Overview of efforts to prevent motor-vehicle-related injury. In *Prevention of motor-vehicle-related injuries: A compendium of articles from the* Morbidity and Mortality Weekly Report, *1985–1996*. Atlanta, GA: U.S. Department of Health and Human Services, Centers for Disease Control and Prevention, National Center for Injury Prevention and Control.

Bunker, J. P., Frazier, H.S., & Mosteller, F. (1994). Improving health: Measuring effects of medical care. *Milbank Quarterly*, *72*, 225–258.

Burt, B. A., & Eklund, S. A. (1999). *Dentistry, dental practice, and the community* (pp. 204–220). Philadelphia: W. B. Saunders.

Centers for Disease Control and Prevention. (1998). Fatal occupational injuries—United States, 1980–1994. *Morbidity and Mortality Weekly Report*, *47*, 297–302.

Centers for Disease Control and Prevention. (1999, April 2). Ten great public health achievements—United States, 1900–1999. *Morbidity and Mortality Weekly Report*, *48*(12), 241–243.

Healthy People 2010, The Office of Disease Prevention and Health Promotion http://www.health.gov/healthypeople/LHI.

Mokdad, A. H., Marks, J. S., Stroup, D. F., et. al. (2004). Actual causes of death in the United States, 2000. *Journal of the American Medical Association*, *291*,1238–1245.

National Center for Health Statistics. (2005). *Health, United States, 2005: With chartbook on trends in the health of Americans.* Hyattsville, MD: Author.

Public Health Service. (1994). *For a healthy nation: Returns on investment in public health.* Atlanta, GA: U.S. Department of Health and Human Services, Public Health Service, Office of Disease Prevention and Health Promotion and Centers for Disease Control and Prevention.

World Health Organization. (1946). Definition of health, Preamble to the Constitution of the World Health Organization, as adopted by the International Health Conference. New York: Author.

World Health Organization, Europe. (1986). *Healthy cities: Promoting health in the urban context.* Copenhagen, Denmark: Author. Retrieved from http://www.euro.who.int/

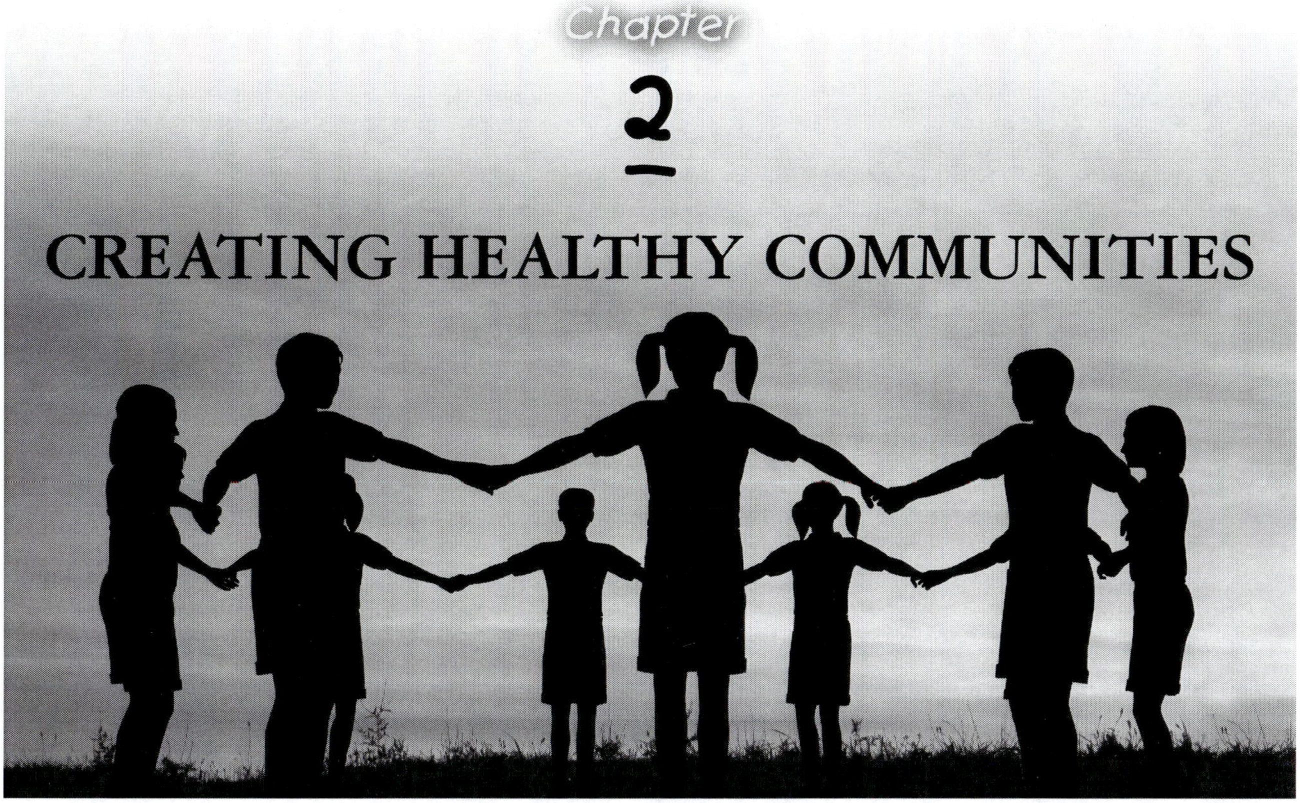

"People who seem to have no power, whether working people, people of color, or women—once they organize and create movements—have a voice no government can suppress."

—Howard Zinn, A People's History of the United States

A Healthy Community Defined

A healthy community is one in which people come together to make their city or town better for themselves, their family, their friends, their neighbors, and others in their community. They share the belief that health is more than merely an absence of disease but includes those elements that enable people to maintain a high quality of life. The community offers access to health-care services that focus on both treatment and prevention for all members of the community.

A healthy community not only offers a physical environment that is safe and clean—including roads, schools, and playgrounds—but also has a high degree of public participation. The participation by community members ensures that basic needs such as food, water, shelter, safety, and work and income are met not only for those who are able to participate but also for those members of the community who—for whatever reason—are unable to participate in the planning and providing of services. The community as a whole has a high positive health status and a low disease status. Community members are able to create and maintain an ongoing dialogue that embraces diversity and fosters a sense of community.

Outlook for Community Health in the 21st Century

The United States' plan for health of Americans is called *Healthy People 2010*. Healthy People 2010 is a set of health objectives that the nation is supposed to have achieved by the end of the first decade of the new century. The two primary goals of this plan were spelled out as follows:

- **Goal 1: Increase quality and years of healthy life.**

The first goal of Healthy People 2010 is to help individuals of all ages increase life expectancy and improve their quality of life.

- **Goal 2: Eliminate health disparities.**

  The second goal of Healthy People 2010 is to eliminate health disparities among different segments of the population.

As a group, "the leading health indicators" presented in the following list reflect the major health concerns in the United States at the beginning of the 21st century. They were designed to measure the health of the nation over the first 10 years of the 21st century and were selected for the following reasons. It was felt that these concerns were relevant enough to motivate action, that data were available to measure progress, and that the indicators were important public health issues. Each of the indicators is presented with an action step, that is, to *promote, prevent, reduce*, and/or *increase* a desired response.

The Leading Health Indicators

1. **Physical activity:** Promote regular physical activity.
2. **Overweight and obesity:** Promote healthier weight and good nutrition.
3. **Tobacco use:** Prevent and reduce tobacco use.
4. **Substance abuse:** Prevent and reduce substance abuse.
5. **Responsible sexual behavior:** Promote responsible sexual behavior.
6. **Mental health:** Promote mental health and well-being.
7. **Injury and violence:** Promote safety and reduce violence.
8. **Environmental quality:** Promote healthy environments.
9. **Immunization:** Prevent infectious disease through immunization.
10. **Access to health care:** Increase access to quality health care.

Health-Promotion Planning and Community Organizing

Organized health-care consumers and communities are engaged throughout the country in a wide range of work to improve health-care access and quality of care, to expand public health, and to reform the health-care system. Their main focus is on (1) obtaining coverage for the uninsured, (2) increasing access to services at the local level, and (3) improving public health.

Among the most important skills is the ability to plan a community health-promotion/disease-prevention program. The actions and conditions that protect and improve community or population health can be organized into three areas: health promotion, health protection, and health services.

Health Promotion

Health promotion is defined as educational and social efforts designed to help people take greater control of and improve their health. It seeks to activate local organizations and groups or individuals to make changes in lifestyle behaviors, participation in community or political action, and in policies that influence health.

Two areas in which communities employ health-promotion strategies are (1) mental and social health, and (2) recreation and fitness. Though both of these health concerns seem to be problems of individuals, a health concern becomes a community or population health concern when many people begin to get sick from specific lifestyle conditions. For example, eating fast food—although an individual activity—can lead to heart disease or diabetes. These chronic diseases can then become public health problems for which public tax money is spent caring for people who are sick with what are considered to be lifestyle and preventable diseases.

Action to deal with these concerns begins with a *community assessment*, which is designed to identify the factors that influence the health of the subpopulations and the needs of these populations. Three approaches to prevention can then be implemented based on the needs of the assessment.

The first approach, **primary prevention**, has the goal of preventing disease from ever occurring. It includes measures that eliminate or forestall the onset of illness. Activities can include exercising or attending meditation classes that enhance nutritional, physical, and mental health.

Secondary prevention is the second approach and involves early diagnosis and prompt intervention or treatment. The goal is to reduce the severity of disease, thereby preventing disability and/or death. This could include the detection of a bacterial respiratory infection and a subsequent prescription of antibiotics.

The third approach, **tertiary prevention**, includes measures aimed at rehabilitation following significant pathogenesis. The goal is to reduce impairment and minimize suffering. Tertiary prevention might take the form of providing rehabilitation services to people involved in an accident.

Health protection and services include the implementing of laws, rules, or policies approved in a community as a result of health promotion or legislation. An example of health protection would be a law to restrict the use of trans fat in food; an example of health services would be a policy offering free condoms by a local health department. Both of these actions could be the result of a *health-promotion effort* such as community members undertaking a letter-writing campaign or lobbying their board of health.

Community Organizing

Community organizing brings people together to combat shared problems and increase their decision-making power. Community organization can be described as an *intervention* in which individuals, groups, and organizations engage in planned action to influence social problems. It can enrich and even develop or change social institutions.

Community organization—not something new to the 21st century—can be seen in events or movements that shaped society as we know it today. When 250,000 people descended on Washington, D.C., to register their support for the *civil rights movement*, they were taken seriously. The Voting Rights Act and desegregation were precipitated by boycotts of businesses and buses in the South—again, in the interest of *civil rights*.

Labor unions were also the result of some pretty impressive community organizing. Until the early 1900s, people often worked long hours for low wages. In 1911, a fire broke out at the Triangle Shirtwaist Company on New York's lower east side, and about 150 employees, almost all of them young women, died. The fire swept through the upper floors of the loft building, killing the workers who were unable to get out of the burning building because the safety exits had been locked to prevent the workers from leaving their workstations. Strikes against conditions in factories throughout the early part of that century led to the 40-hour work week and better working conditions for all workers.

The *feminist movement* brought about important changes not only in voting rights but also in health care. The "community" of women fought for equal rights, which resulted in the right to vote; equal pay for equal work; the right to initiate divorce; and the right of women to make individual decisions regarding pregnancy, including obtaining contraceptives and safe abortions. In health care, the movement successfully challenged the medical model of childbirth, helped make breast-feeding an important preventive measure, and made domestic violence a public health issue.

More recently, gay organizations and—in the last several years—organizations in communities of color have made an impact in *health movements*. These movements have addressed AIDS treatment and organization of care, discrimination, drug policy, research, public health programs, and the role of the consumer.

As can be seen in the preceding examples, *community organizing* occurs when people form their own organizations to provide long-term capacity for problem solving. We describe three basic types of community organizing before moving on to the actual process of program planning.

Grassroots organizing builds community groups from scratch, develops new leadership where none existed, and otherwise organizes the unorganized. The term *grassroots* is alleged to have been started by Senator Albert Jeremiah Beveridge of Indiana who said, speaking of the Progressive Party in 1912, "This party has come from the grass roots. It has grown from the soil of people's hard necessities."

Faith-based community organizing (FBCO) develops power and relationships throughout a community of institutions. This community of institutions can include groups such as congregations, unions, and associations.

The third type of community organizing results in the formation of a *coalition.* A **coalition** is an *alliance* among entities, during which they cooperate in *joint action*, each in their own *self-interest*. This alliance may be temporary or a matter of convenience. It is merely the coming together of individuals or groups who have common interests and who stand to benefit individually from the coalition.

> ***"A single bracelet does not jingle."***
>
> ***—African proverb***

The Process of Program Planning

Program planning is a process by which an intervention is planned to help meet the needs of a target population. Assessing the needs of the target population is the first task in creating a health-promotion/disease-prevention program. Recall that we introduced the *community assessment* earlier in this chapter in terms of establishing prevention plans. You need to know the community in which you will be working and the history of the specific issue or issues you will address. Allow ample time for your group to become familiar with the community, its history, makeup, demographics, geography, and political leadership. At this time, you will be determining who the people are that your group needs to interview and the questions you want to ask. If members of your group are not already members of the community and "in the know," community members are your best resources for helping you to gain entry. Not only civic volunteers but also health-care providers and people who work in human/social services are likely to know what needs are most pressing. Other options include workers from grassroots agencies; people who are involved in recreation or parks programs; and, of course, education and government employees. Depending on the nature of your purpose in organizing, you may also wish to speak to community people involved in neighborhood associations, faith-based organizations, businesses, media, and/or law enforcement.

One-on-one interviews—the main goals of which are to listen and gather information—are an important part of community organizing. "Organizers" or "planners" should try to first meet with people individually rather than trying to meet everyone in a group setting. After gathering data—again, the prime reason for the interviews—time is spent analyzing the data and prioritizing (organizing) identified needs, which then need to be verified or validated.

Based on your initial assessment and interviews, the foundation for your program is laid by setting goals and objectives.

> **Goals:** The general statements that describe the desired solution to a problem or issue.
>
> **Objectives:** The specific statements that describe the changes expected to achieve a goal. Objectives are usually written as subsets to goals, which means that two or more objectives may be associated with a single goal. Goals describe in broad terms what the program will achieve. *Example:* The overall goal of a school-based health-control effort should be to reduce infections and prevent re-infections among students and school staff.

Planning the goals of the program requires the establishment of both outcome objectives and process objectives. The delineation of both types of objectives helps to ensure that all participants understand what actions must be taken, why, when, and what measure of success these actions are achieving.

An **outcome objective** defines and describes what the outcome of a particular action is intended to achieve, and it does so in concrete, measurable ways. Recall that one of the criteria for determining the leading health indicators is that there will be data available for measuring progress. Outcome objectives for the program include the specific steps intended to improve the health status of participants in the program, as well as changes in their understanding, attitudes, beliefs, behaviors, and conditions related to the problem that the goal is intended to solve; that is, outcome objectives define what conditions will exist if the program is successful.

- Example of outcome objective: *By 2013, the number of children who have the flu will be reduced by 10%.*

A **process objective** defines a specific step that will be implemented in the process of attempting to achieve the outcome objectives.

- Example of process objective: *By 2010, the number of schools in Bayside that have implemented flu-reduction interventions will have increased from 15 to 18.*

Developing an intervention involves actually designing the activities that will help target population members meet their objectives. Work with your team to develop an intervention. What problems has your group identified? What policies would address that problem? What decision-making body do you need to impact? What other steps will your team need to take to change policy? Break your work down into manageable steps and tasks. Include a time line for when things will happen and identify who is responsible for what. The time line should be realistic and feasible and, above all, flexible.

Implementing the intervention is actually putting into practice the activities that made up the intervention. Once you achieve your goal, your group will need to decide how it will maintain the change to ensure that the desired results are achieved. You wil also have to decide what the future of the planning group will be once you attain your goal. Has the group served its purpose? Do you want to work on other policies?

After the intervention has been implemented and the campaign is over, **evaluate**. *Evaluating the results* is comparing the program's outcome with some standard of acceptability that was noted in the goals and objectives. As you implement your plan of action, it is important to carefully review your progress during the intervention. Steps in the evaluation process are similar to the steps in the information-gathering process:

1. Plan the evaluation.
2. Collect the data.
3. Analyze the data.
4. Report results.
5. Apply the results.

Following are some examples of evaluation questions to ask leaders and other stakeholders in your campaign.

- Is the campaign making a difference? How?
- Are we making progress toward our goal?
- What factors are most important in achieving the goals of the campaign?
- What are the biggest challenges or obstacles for the campaign?
- What has been accomplished?
- What still needs to be done?
- What was done well?
- What could have been done better?

Activism, Advocacy, and Empowerment

Some important terms that are especially relevant in establishing health-care programs are *activism, advocacy*, and *empowerment.* **Activism** refers to individuals first taking responsibility for their own health care, working toward the improvement of health conditions for a specific community, and making efforts to change and improve policies and standards that affect large populations.

Advocacy is action taken in support of a particular cause. Health advocacy is often political, because it tends to focus on changes in legislation and other forms of policy or funding allocations.

Empowerment refers to the feeling of power and control over our own lives; this empowerment results from the time, energy, and resources we dedicate to improving health problems. Empowerment can exist at four levels: (1) the personal level, by gaining control and influence in daily life and in community participation; (2) the small-group level, through the shared experience, analysis, and influence of small groups on their own efforts; (3) the organizational level, through capacity building by influencing decision-making processes; and (4) the community level, by gaining and utilizing resources and strategies to enhance community control.

Being Proactive As—or On Behalf of—a Patient

Hopefully, it is clear that activism, advocacy, and empowerment are important pieces of being community minded. Likewise, being **proactive** is just as important. Taking a *proactive* stance as—or on behalf of—a patient involves the following:

- Know patient rights.
- Find out about informed consent procedures, living wills, durable power of attorney, organ donation, and other legal issues *before* you become sick or find yourself in the position of needing the information for someone else.
- Ask about alternative procedures.
- If a loved one (friend or relative) is the patient, remain with your loved one as a personal advocate.
- Monitor the actions of health-care providers.
- Be considerate of care providers.
- Be patient with the patient. (This includes being patient with yourself if you are the patient.)

The relationship between patients and their physicians should be viewed as a partnership in which communication is central. Making decisions about health care is becoming a shared, communicative process between patients and their providers. Providers must be sensitive to patients' beliefs and cultural values when collaborating about health decisions.

To be a *proactive patient*, an individual should obtain—or attempt to obtain—increased knowledge about his or her own health problems. This will involve assertiveness and the willingness to participate in informed decisions regarding his or her health.

Proactive individuals must take some responsibility for coordinating their own health information so that it is accessible and so that they can better understand their own health histories. *Self-advocacy* is representing one's own interests within a health-care decision-making process. Healthy citizens engage in their own self-advocacy by being their own advocates by asking key questions, searching for information, and ensuring proper care.

The terms *public advocacy and health activism* refer to the efforts of groups with common health concerns to have their voices heard and needs met through prioritization of vital issues, various forms of interpersonal and mass media, and participation in national decision-making processes. Recall that many of the definitions we have discussed in this chapter have included the ability to increase decision making as part of the process. Through grassroots methods of advocacy, organizations such as Mothers Against Drunk Driving (MADD) have made great strides in raising public awareness about drunk driving, promoting research, and influencing legislation.

Example of an Advocacy Campaign: "Agenda for a Healthy New York"

New York City faces serious health challenges. Rates of type 2 diabetes are increasing and half of New Yorkers are overweight or obese. Additionally, more than a quarter of New Yorkers under the age of 65 lack health insurance. Health disparities along racial and socioeconomic lines have also increased which cause inequities in health between the rich and poor and between racial and ethnic minorities. The widening gap of diabetes, the infant mortality rate in low income neighborhoods being double that in wealthier areas, and the fact that African American women are 7 times more likely than white women to die of pregnancy-related causes serve as evidence of profound racial and socioeconomic health disparities.

Did you know?

1 in 4 New Yorkers does not exercise

1 in 5 New Yorkers is obese

1 in 8 New Yorkers has diabetes

2 in 5 NYC public elementary school children are overweight

Examples of Policy Interventions to Achieve a Healthy New York:

Increase the availability and affordability of healthy foods including fruits, vegetables, whole grains and low fat dairy products.

- Eliminate soda, candy, and foods high in fat and sugar from all NYC public schools and promote 1% milk, water, fresh fruits and vegetables, and whole grain breads;
- Increase access to healthy food by expanding farmers markets and promoting new relationships among local agricultural producers and institutional, commercial and individual consumers;
- Facilitate enrollment for those eligible for Food Stamps by simplifying the application form and by making it available online and at food distribution sites.

Increase opportunities for physical activity.

- Enforce state mandates for physical education in city schools;
- Create and improve safe and accessible public spaces such as playgrounds, city parks, public schools, and walking and recreation areas;
- Develop workplace physical activity programs for all city workers.

Increase access to preventive reproductive and sexual health care.

- Expand the availability of pregnancy-prevention counseling and contraception including emergency contraception and condoms at community organizations, hospitals, health clinics, and high schools;
- Conduct intensive outreach on prenatal care and contraceptive use to high risk groups and increase the capacity of home visiting programs to serve more pregnant women and new parents;
- Fully fund existing and develop new reimbursement mechanisms in New York State to support the work of reproductive health providers who provide women's wellness services and to allow for increased enrollment.

Reduce the barriers to getting timely and effective primary and preventive care.

- Develop comprehensive city-wide programs for management and control of asthma and diabetes;
- Provide financial support to community health efforts in NYC, and expand and improve services centers;
- Oppose state and federal cuts to Medicaid that reduce access to primary and preventive care.

Source: PHANYC 2005, Agenda for Healthy New York.

References

Daniel, M., & Green, L. W. (1999). Community-based prevention and chronic disease self-management programmes: Problems, praises and pitfalls. *Disease Management and Health Outcomes, 6*(4), 185–192.

Flynn, B. C., Ray, D. W., & Rider, M. S. (1994). Empowering communities: Action research through healthy cities. *Health Education Quarterly*, *21*, 395–406.

Frankish, C. J., & Green, L. W. (1994). Organizational and community change as the basis for disease prevention and health promotion policy. *Advances in Medical Sociology, 4*, 209–233.

Green, L. W. (1978). Determining the impact and effectiveness of health education as it relates to federal policy. *Health Education Monographs, 6*, 28–66.

Green, L. W., & Kreuter, M. W. (1999). *Health promotion planning: An educational and ecological approach* (3rd ed.). Mountain View, CA: Mayfield Publishing.

Green, L. W., & Ottoson, J. M. (1999). *Community and population health* (8th ed.). Boston: WCB/McGraw-Hill.

Kreuter, M. W., Lezin, N. A., Kreuter, M. W., & Green, L. W. (1998). *Community health promotion ideas that work: A field-book for practitioners.* Boston: Jones and Bartlett.

Lee, P. R., & Estes, C. L. (1997). *The nation's health* (5th ed.). Boston: Jones and Bartlett.

Mausner, J. S., & Kramer, S. (1985). *Epidemiology: An introductory text.* Philadelphia: W. B. Saunders.

McKenzie, J. F., Pinger, R. R., & Kotecki, J. E. (1999). *An introduction to community health* (3rd ed.). Boston: Jones and Bartlett.

McKenzie, J. F., & Smeltzer, J. L. (1997). *Planning, implementing, and evaluating health promotion programs: A primer* (2nd ed.). Boston: Allyn & Bacon.

Miller, D. F., & Price, J. H. (1998). *Dimensions of community health* (5th ed.). Boston: WCB/McGraw-Hill.

Pickett, G., & Hanlon, J. J. (1990). *Public health: Administration and practice* (9th ed.). St. Louis, MO: Times Mirror/Mosby, Inc.

Rosen, G. (1993). *A history of public health.* Baltimore: Johns Hopkins University Press.

Rubin, H. J., & Rubin, I. S. (1992). *Community organizing and development* (2nd ed.). New York: Macmillan.

Turnock, B. J. (1997). *Public health: What it is and how it works.* Gaithersburg, MD: Aspen Publishers.

U.S. Department of Health and Human Services, Public Health Service. (1991). *Healthy people 2000: National health promotion and disease prevention objectives* (DHHS Publication No. [PHS] 91–50212). Washington, DC: Author.

Chapter

3

PREVENTION AND CONTROL OF DISEASES

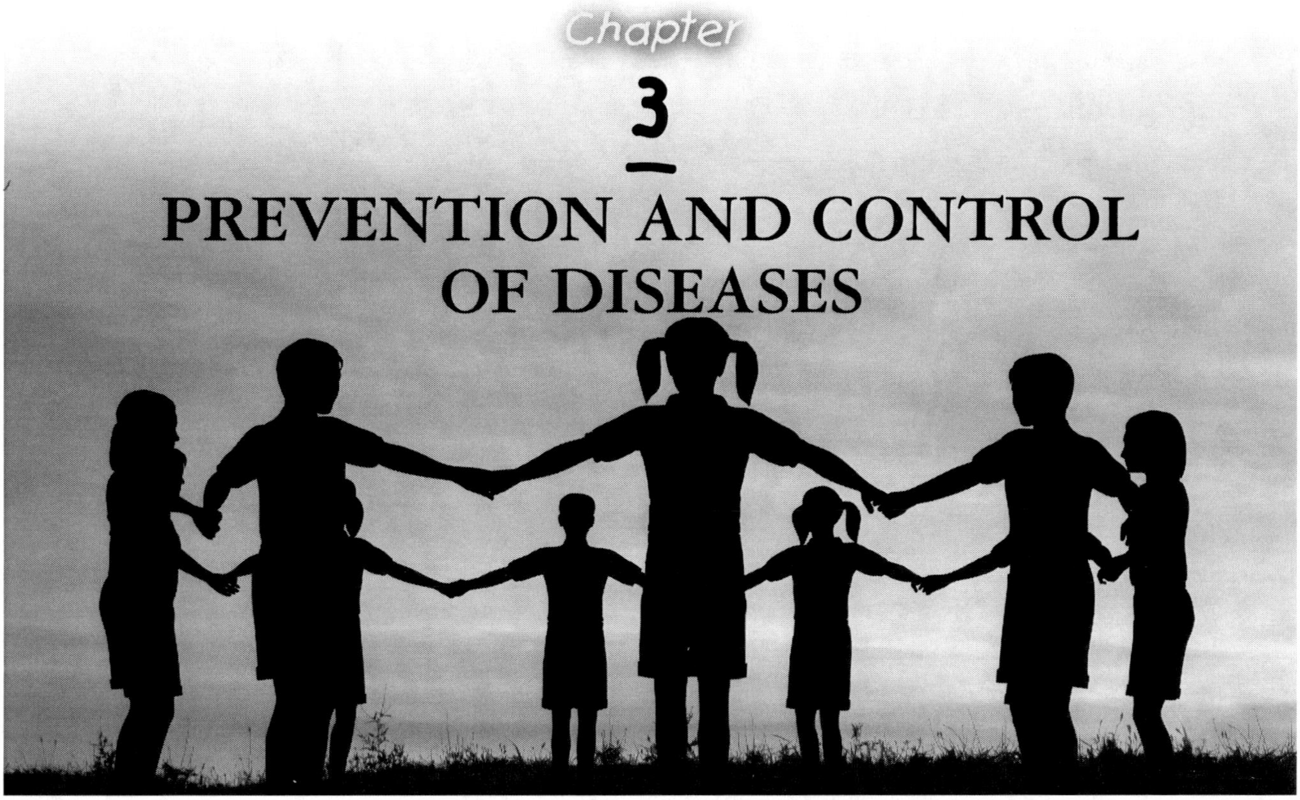

"Every human being is the author of his or her own health or disease."

—Hindu Prince Guatama Siddhartha, founder of Buddahism

Community health education is designed to promote health and prevent disease within populations. People who study community health use their theoretical knowledge to develop and implement programs that are intended to maintain health and prevent diseases to the extent possible for specific populations in a community.

Community health efforts have a three-pronged approach: epidemiology, community organization, and health education.

Epidemiology

Epidemiology is a branch of medicine that involves the study of the causes, distribution, and control of disease in populations. Its focus is on the factors that affect both the health and illness of populations.

An **epidemiologist** might work on a wide range of issues, including investigations related to outbreaks of diseases and environmental exposure to toxins; the general promotion of health; and the development of biological, statistical, and psychosocial theories regarding disease. Important aspects of the work of epidemiologists include identifying and defining diseases, making causational connections between and among diseases, and formulating effective strategies for health.

It is important to note that epidemics of communicable diseases have commonly existed throughout human history, and that epidemiologists have played a significant role in identifiying and controlling such diseases.

Pioneers of Epidemiology

Anton van Leeuwenhoek (1632–1723) is considered the father of microscopy, having been the first person to create a practical microscope with which he was able to view bacteria.

Louis Pasteur convinced the medical world of the concept of viruses, or germs, proved that certain diseases are caused by infectious agents, and developed the process of pasteurization and a vaccine for rabies.

Jonas Salk and Albert Sabin created successful vaccines for smallpox and polio, respectively.

Alexander Fleming discovered the first antibiotic penicillin.

Gerhard Domagk developed sulphonamides, the first synthetic antibiotic that could be used for a broad spectrum of bacterial infections.

Dr. John Snow supressed the 1854 outbreak of cholera in London's Soho district by identifying the fact that the disease was contracted through contaminated water at specific locations.

British surgeon Joseph Lister, based upon Pasteur's earlier work, in 1865, introduced the concept of antiseptic methods in surgery.

Major Premise of Epidemiology:

Diseases and illnesses do not randomly occur within a population; instead, there are specific causes and solutions.

Objectives of Epidemiology:

1. Identify the causes of specific diseases and the factors that increase a person's risk of those diseases.
2. Identify the extent of diseases that exist in a community.
3. Identify and explain the natural history and characteristics of specific diseases.
4. Evaluate preventive and therapeutic measures to prevent diseases.
5. Provide input into policy decisions that are made within communities.

Epidemiological Studies

Descriptive studies investigate the extent of disease outbreaks as they relate to people, places, and time periods.

Analytical studies test theories and hypotheses about the relationships between health problems and possible risk factors.

Retrospective studies compare people with diseases (experimental test cases) to healthy people of similar ages, genders, and backgrounds (control groups), regarding previous exposure to possible risk factors.

Prospective studies classify subjects that belong to a large group of people with similar experiences and have similar exposures to specific risk factors, and they are observed ongoingly to identify any possible disease outcomes.

Experimental studies are designed to identify causes of diseases and the efficacy of treatments for such diseases. This is accomplished by controlling the greatest number of variables related to the experimental subjects. Typically, experimental studies adhere to the standard principles of using control groups, randomization, and giving no knowledge to the researchers or participants of the details of the studies until after the data have been recorded.

1. Control groups receive a placebo instead if a drug, which, unbeknownst to them, is not in a treatment at all.
2. Those who participate in experimental studies are assigned to control and treatment groups randomly.
3. With professional experiments, both subjects and researchers remain uninformed about the identity of treatment and control groups until after the data have been recorded.

The Importance of Rates

Rates are the occurrences and spread of diseases in populations. Rates car ıssessed in several different ways, including for a specific group of people and for an entire country's populati uch rates are used for national purposes as health indicators, which include **life expectancy**, or how long pe an expect to live; **infant mortality**, or how many infants die before they reach age one; and the major caus death and the amount and types of illnesses in a national population. A common rate is the number of de caused by specific diseases. When the national death rate for a certain disease is high, this can be a warning serious health issue.

The following are major types of rates of disease within a populatior

An **incidence rate** is the number of new cases of a disease ir pulation-at-risk in a specific time period divided by the number of people in the population.

A **prevalence rate** is the number of new and old cases of a se occurring in a specific time period divided by number of people in the population.

An **attack rate** is a special incidence rate calculated for a cular population for a single outbreak of a disease and expressed as a percent.

Mortality and Morbidity

Mortality is a measure of the incidences of deaths in a p ation. Reporting deaths is a legal requirement that is supported by a national data collection system. A sudd crease in deaths resulting from the same causes in one geographic region can alert health officials to an envi ental problem, such as a water-borne disease outbreak.

Morbidity is a measure of the number of people wh e contracted a disease during a specific time period (**incidence rate**) or the number of people who current e that disease (**prevalence rate**) in relation to the size of the population. Morbidity can suggest connectior ween current health conditions and possible environmental factors in the analysis of trends in diseases and id ying factors that cause specific diseases.

The Reporting of Births, Deaths, and Dise ccurs in Four Steps:

1. Births, deaths, and cases of certain di s that occur in the United States must be reported to health authorities.
2. Local health departments are requir summarize all records of births, deaths, and diseases and report them to their state health departm
3. Local state health departments th rn over the reports to the Centers for Disease Control (CDC).
4. Local, state, and federal govern s maintain vital and disease records, which are used by health professionals to track and study dise

Factors That Aff a Country's Mortality Rate

- the average age of a country' ulation
- nutrition levels
- standards of diet and ho
- access to clean drinkin er
- hygiene levels
- levels of infectious d es
- levels of violent cr

- conflicts
- the number of doctors

Infant Mortality Rate

Infant mortality and life expectancy are two key indicators of any nation's overall health. The major causes of infant mortality throughout the world are pneumonia, dehydration from diarrhea, and malnutrition resulting from poverty and unsafe food and water. The main causes of infant mortality in developed countries are infections and SIDS.

U.S. Infant Mortality Is Among the Worst in Industrialized Nations

The rate of infant mortality in the United States is higher than those of many other developed countries. Among thirty-three industrialized nations, the United States is tied with Hungary, Malta, Poland, and Slovakia with an infant mortality rate of nearly 5 per 1,000 infants. Japan had the lowest rate, 1.8 deaths per 1,000 infants.

The high infant mortality in the United States is partially a result of portions of the population with low incomes. Also, the population of the United States is much more racially, as well as economically, diverse than other industrialized countries, which creates a challenge to provide culturally appropriate health care. Among African Americans, the infant mortality rate is 9 deaths per 1,000 infants, which is closer to rates in developing countries than to those in developed countries. About half a million U.S. babies are born prematurely each year. African-American infants are twice as likely as are white infants to be born prematurely, to have low birth weights, and to die at birth.

Possible factors that contribute to the high infant mortality rates in the U.S. include the following:

- high rates of teen pregnancies
- high rates of obesity
- the lack of national universal health insurance
- short maternity leaves
- poor access to health care
- poverty and discrimination

All of these factors can contribute to a woman's poor health care before and during pregnancy, thus increasing the risk of premature birth and low birth weight, the leading causes of newborn death in developed countries. The least-developed nations account for 99 percent of the 4 million deaths per year of infants in their first month, mainly as a result of infections. The highest rates are in Africa and South Asia.

Classification of Diseases and Health Problems

Diseases and health problems can be classified in several meaningful ways.

A **communicable disease** is an infectious disease that can be transmitted from one person or species to another. Communicable diseases are spread through direct contact with an infected person or through contact with bodily fluids or objects that infected persons have touched.

An **infectious disease** is a disease that damages or harms the host. Infectious diseases result from the presence of microbial agents, including viruses, bacteria, fungi, protozoa, multicellular parasites, and prions (infectious proteins). People with low-income, women, children, and the elderly are most vulnerable to infectious diseases, which continue to be the world's leading cause of death of young adults and children.

Infectivity is the ability of an organism to enter, survive, and multiply in a host.

Infectiousness is the ease with which a disease is transmitted to other hosts.

An **infection** is different from an infectious disease in that an infection might not cause symptoms or impair the functions of the host.

The World Health Organization (WHO) collects data about global deaths by International Classification of Disease (ICD) code categories.

Top Infectious Diseases Worldwide:

1. Lower respiratory infections
2. HIV/AIDS
3. Diarrheal diseases
4. Tuberculosis (TB)
5. Malaria
6. Measles
7. Pertussis
8. Tetanus
9. Meningitis
10. Syphilis

*(Source: **World Health Organization** at www.who.int/whosis/icd10/)*

How Infections Spread

Infection is a chain of transmission of a communicable disease from one source to a new, susceptible host. For an infection to occur, each link in this chain of transmission must be present and in sequential order. The links are as follows: an infectious agent, a reservoir, a portal of exiting the reservoir, a mode of transmission, and a portal of entry into a susceptible host. An awareness of this cycle also provides knowledge of methods of self-protection.

An **Infectious Agent** is a microbial organism that can cause disease. Infectious agents include bacteria, virus, fungi, and parasites.

- **Bacteria:** Bacteria are unicellular organisms. They multiply by dividing themselves into new bacteria. Bacteria exist everywhere, including inside and on humans' bodies. Some bacteria live in the intestines and help boost the immune system. These are referred to as "good" bacteria. To maintain a healthy level of good bacteria, people must take in probiotics or eat yogurt that contains active live cultures. On the other hand, people sometimes need to take antibiotics to kill harmful bacteria. Antibiotics kill not only the bad bacteria, however, but also the good bacteria. The overuse of antibiotics has caused bacteria today to be more resistant to these drugs and therefore they are more difficult to kill.
- **Viruses:** Unlike bacteria, viruses cannot multiply by themselves, so they must invade a host cell and take over its function to be able to create new viral cells. Viruses are made of genetic material (DNA or RNA) surrounded by a protective protein coat. Viruses can invade cells, and once they do, they take over the cells and reproduce new viral cells. The host cells usually die after the reproduction of new viral cells. RNA viruses are unstable and thus often mutate. DNA viruses are more stable; thus, they mutate less often than do RNA viruses. A retrovirus is a type of RNA virus that invades the body's cells, where it produces more such RNA viruses: includes the AIDS virus and many cancer-causing viruses (leukemia).

Antibiotics are ineffective against viruses, such as colds and flu's. Thus, it is important for people to limit the use of antibiotics only to bacterial infections. Again, the overuse of antibiotics decreases their effectiveness by encouraging the growth of antibiotic-resistant bacteria, which has become an increasingly serious worldwide problem.

A **reservoir** is a place in which microorganisms live and reproduce. Microorganisms thrive within the bodies of humans and animals, as well as in water and on tabletops and doorknobs.

A **portal of exit** is a place from which microorganisms leave a reservoir. An example of a microorganism leaving a portal of exit is when they are expelled through the nose or mouth when a person sneezes or coughs.

A **mode of transmission** is a method by which an organism travels from one infected individual or group to a previously uninfected individual or group. Modes of transmission can be direct or indirect. **Direct transmission** includes touching (including through sexual contact), coughing, and sneezing. **Indirect transmission** can be airborne, vehicle-borne or vector-borne.

The following are definitions of different modes of disease transmission:

- **droplet contact:** coughing or sneezing on another person
- **direct physical contact:** touching an infected person, including sexual contact
- **indirect contact:** touching a contaminated surface, including, in some cases, soil
- **airborne transmission:** occurs when a microorganism can remain in the air for a long period of time
- **fecal-oral transmission:** often occurs from contaminated food or water sources
- **vector-borne transmission:** the carrying of disease by insects or other animals

The Role of Humans in the Transmission of Diseases

The construction of new housing developments in previously uninhabited areas brings people into contact with animals and thus with the microbes that they harbor as well. In Florida, for example, many swamplands are being destroyed to make way for new construction of homes, but the alligators, as well as the microbes associated with them, remain in the vicinity, and eventually, these microbes can be transmitted to people. This type of disease transmission also occurs in the rain forests that are being cut down.

Disease transmission to and by humans also results when the rapid growth of cities, particularly in developing countries, forces large numbers of people into crowded areas with poor sanitation. In addition, global warming changes ecosystems in ways that move microbes into new areas.

A **portal of entry** is an opening in which a microorganism is able to enter the body of a host. Some portals of entry include body orifices, mucus membranes, and cuts in the skin.

A **susceptible host** is a body that a microorganism can invade, multiply, and cause an infection.

Disease Control

A major goal of public health is to prevent the spread of infectious diseases in populations and to contain outbreaks when they do occur. Vaccines are a primary means of preventing diseases in people who receive them. Vaccines prevent and control many infectious diseases that were once common in the United States, including polio, mumps, measles, diphtheria, tetanus, pertussis (whooping cough), rubella (German measles), and *Haemophilus influenzae* type b (Hib).

(Source: Centers for Disease Control)

What is a vaccine?

A vaccine exposes a person to germs in a controlled manner. A vaccine contains dead or weakened germs that cause a specific type of disease. When a person is vaccinated, his or her body reacts by creating protective substances called antibodies, which defend the body by helping to kill the germs that enter the body. The person does not contract the particular disease but is then protected from it.

Like a real disease, a vaccine creates **active immunity** because the body has a lasting memory of the infection. **Passive immunity** is acquired through breast milk or immunoglobulin shots given for allergies. Passive immunity lasts for only a few months. **Herd immunity** is the protection not just of a vaccinated person but also of others who come in contact with that person. Through herd immunity, it is sometimes possible to completely **eradicate** an infection, which occurs when there is no risk of infection or disease anywhere in the world. So far, the only infectious disease that has been eradicated is smallpox, the last case of which occurred in 1979. However, because several laboratories kept samples of the smallpox virus, it is not actually extinct. **Extinction** occurs when an agent no longer exists in nature or in a laboratory.

Prevention of Disease

Prevention is taking action to avert the onset of a disease before it is contracted. **Intervention** is taking action to control a disease in progress. **Control** is the containment of a disease and can include both prevention and intervention. Prevention is clearly the best means of controlling a disease.

Levels of Prevention

- **Primary prevention** is averting an illness before the disease process can begin (e.g., education).
- **Secondary prevention** is the early diagnosis and immediate treatment of a disease before it becomes advanced and disability becomes severe (e.g., screening).
- **Tertiary prevention** is the retraining, reeducating, and rehabilitating of a person who has already contracted and is suffering from a disease (e.g., emergency medical services).

Breaking the Cycle of Infection

Preventing infection is a matter of examining one's lifestyle choices, habits, and environment, and then assessing which of these areas might lead to infection. By identifying areas in the chain of infection, people can take steps to eliminate them. The following are some basic steps to help prevent infections:

- Practice good personal hygiene. Frequent and proper hand washing is essential in preventing the spread of infection.
  - Always wash your hands (sing the happy birthday song) before handling or eating food.
- Treat all bodily fluids as potentially infectious.
  - Use protective barriers such as gloves, masks, aprons, and condoms when exposure to infectious agents is possible.
- Maintain a clean home and environment.
- Store and cook foods at the proper temperatures.
- Properly dispose of wastes, garbage, and used medical supplies.
- See your doctor regularly for protective vaccines and immunizations.

The Pandemic of Lifestyle Diseases

In the early1900s, the leading causes of death in the United States were communicable diseases such as pneumonia, influenza, tuberculosis, and diarrhea. Since the 1940s, however, the majority of deaths in the United States have resulted from diseases related to lifestyles, such as heart disease and cancer.

Lifestyle diseases are those that result from the ways in which people live: diet, habits, environment, and levels of exercise all play critical roles in the development or nondevelopment of such diseases. Lifestyle diseases are different from other diseases because they are potentially preventable, and the risk of contracting them can be reduced by an awareness in and appropriate changes in diet, lifestyle, habits, and environment.

Many lifestyle diseases are related to obesity and physical inactivity. These include heart disease, type 2 diabetes, Alzheimer's disease, atherosclerosis, asthma, cancer, chronic liver disease or cirrhosis of the liver, chronic obstructive pulmonary disease, metabolic syndrome, nephritis or chronic renal failure, osteoporosis, stroke, and depression.

Communicable versus Noncommunicable Diseases

Noncommunicable diseases cannot be transmitted from one person to another. For example, diseases of the heart and blood vessels are noncommunicable diseases. They are the leading cause of death in the United States.

Communicable diseases are infectious diseases that can be transmitted from one infected person to another, either by direct contact or indirectly.

Examples of Communicable Diseases

Human Influenza (Flu)

Influenza, or the flu, is a contagious respiratory illness caused by influenza viruses. The flu is associated with mild to severe symptoms and illness. It some cases, it can cause death. Every year, between 5% and 20% of the population of the United States contracts the flu. Some people, such as older people, young children, and people with certain health conditions are at a higher risk for serious flu complications, which can include bacterial pneumonia, ear infections, sinus infections, dehydration, and worsening of chronic medical conditions, such as congestive heart failure, asthma, and diabetes. Today, about 250,000 to 500,000 people worldwide die of influenza every year.

(Source: www.cdc.gov/flu/)

A **flu epidemic** occurs when a flu virus spreads rapidly throughout a population. Flu epidemics are common within certain populations nearly every year. In contrast, an **influenza pandemic** is an epidemic of an influenza virus that spreads throughout the world and infects a large percentage of the human population. Unlike the common seasonal epidemics of influenza, pandemics do not occur as often.

Based on historical records, influenza pandemics have most likely occurred during at least the last four centuries. Since the early 1900s, three pandemics and several "pandemic threats" have occurred.

1918–1919: The Spanish Flu. The worst flu pandemic recorded was the Spanish flu of 1918–1919, which killed an estimated 50 million people worldwide and 500,000 in the United States alone. This pandemic is the catastrophe against which all modern pandemics are measured. An estimated 20% to 40% of the world's population became ill from the Spanish flu, and more than 50 million people died as a result. Between September of 1918 and April of 1919, approximately 675,000 deaths from the flu occurred in the United States alone. Many people who contracted the flu died from it quickly. Many others died several days or weeks later of complications resulting from the flu (such as pneumonia). One of the most unique aspects of the Spanish flu was its ability to kill young adults.

(Source: http://1918.pandemicflu.gov/)

1957: The Asian Flu. The Asian influenza pandemic began in 1957 in Asia. Unlike the Spanish flu virus that caused the 1918–1919 pandemic, the Asian flu virus was quickly detected (in February of 1957) as a result of advances in scientific and medical technology. Vaccines became available in limited supply by August of 1957. The virus spread to the United States quietly, with a series of small, isolated outbreaks during the summer of 1957. However, when children went back to school in the fall, they spread the virus there and then at home to their families. About 69,800 people in the United States died from the Asian flu pandemic, but the highest rates of death were among the elderly.

(Source: http://www.flu.gov/individualfamily/about/)

1968: The Hong Kong Flu. In early 1968, the Hong Kong influenza pandemic was first identified in Hong Kong. People who were older than age 65 were most susceptible to death from the virus. The virus resurfaced in 1970 and 1972. Approximately 1 million people throughout the world died from the Hong Kong flu pandemic, with about 33,800 in the United States.

(Source: http://www.flu.gov)

1997: The Avian Flu Threat. In 1997, several hundred people became infected with the avian A/H5N1 flu virus in Hong Kong. The avian virus was a new kind of virus because it traveled directly from chickens to people. Some of the people most severely affected were young adults. To prevent further spreading of this virus, all of the chickens (approximately 1.5 million) in Hong Kong were killed. The avian flu did not easily spread from one person to another, so after the chickens had been killed, no new human infections were identified.

In 1999, another avian flu virus, A/H9N2, was identified in Hong Kong. Although neither of these two avian viruses became pandemics, their continued presence in poultry, their ability to infect humans, and their capability to change and become more transmissible among people is an ongoing concern for scientists.

(Source: http://www.flu.gov)

***2009: The Swine Flu:** A(H1N1).* The swine flu A(H1N1) originated in Mexico and spread to the United States in April of 2009. It then spread to more than seventy countries around the world. On June 10, 2009, the World Health Organization (WHO) reported 27,737 cases of the swine flue, including 141 deaths. The WHO has stressed that most cases are mild and do not require treatment, but there is a fear that an outbreak of new infections could overwhelm hospitals and health authorities, especially in less-developed countries.

The swine flu is caused by a virus that usually affects pigs, but the A(H1N1) strain is a combination of pig, human, and bird viruses and is transmitted from person to person. On June 11, 2009, the WHO declared a swine flu pandemic—the first global flu epidemic in 41 years. It is especially dangerous in children and young adults.

(Source: http://www.cdc.gov/h1n1flu/)

Symptoms of flu include the following:

- fever
- headache
- extreme tiredness
- dry cough
- sore throat
- runny or stuffy nose
- muscle aches
- stomach symptoms, such as nausea, vomiting, and diarrhea, also can occur, but these are more common in children than adults

Flu viruses typically spread from one person to another through the coughing or sneezing of a person who has influenza or by touching something with a flu virus on it and then touching the mouth or nose. Healthy adults often are able to infect others beginning just one day before symptoms develop and up to five days after becoming ill.

The **flu shot** is an inactivated vaccine, meaning that it contains the dead virus. The flu shot is approved for people age 6 months and older, both for those who are healthy and those who have chronic medical conditions. About two weeks after receiving the flue shot, a person's body develops antibodies that protect against an influenza virus infection.

(Source: www.cdc.gov/flu/about/qa/flushot.htm)

Another form of a vaccination for influenza is in the form of a nasal spray. The nasal-spray flu vaccine, sometimes called LAIV for "Live Attenuated Influenza Vaccine," is made with a live, weakened flu virus. The LAIV is approved for use in healthy people age 5 to 49 years of age who are not pregnant.

People at high risk for complications from the flu include the following:

- children age 6 months to age 5
- pregnant women,
- people 50 years of age and older,
- people of any age with certain chronic medical conditions, such as asthma
- health-care workers
- people who live in nursing homes and other long-term care facilities

(Source: www.cdc.gov/flu/about/disease/symptoms)

CA-MRSA: Methicillin-Resistant *Staphylococcus Aureus*

Staphylococcus aureus is also known as "staph" bacteria. **Staph infections** often begin when the bacteria enter the body through an opening, such as a cut, in the skin. The bacteria are transmitted from the skin of an infected person and onto the skin of another person when they have direct contact. It is also transmitted when an infected person touches items and surfaces, from which the bacteria then enter the skin of other people who touch those items and surfaces.

Staph bacteria are being transmitted to increasing numbers of people, causing serious and sometimes fatal skin infections that are resistant to many antibiotics. These resistant strains of staph, known as "MRSA," can be easily spread in gyms, hospitals and other facilities where people gather together.

Symptoms of a staph skin infection include redness, swelling, blisters, and tenderness of the skin.

The following can help prevent the spread of antibiotic-resistant staph skin infections:

- Keep any infected areas covered with clean, dry bandages.
- Wash your hands often with soap and warm water.
- Regularly clean your bathroom and personal items.
- Do not share razors, towels, or similar personal items with others.

Meningitis

Meningitis is classified into the following categories:

- Meningococcal meningitis is an inflammation of the membranes surrounding the brain and spinal cord.
- Meningococcemia is an infection in the bloodstream.
- Viral meningitis is the most common form of meningitis. It is caused by a virus, not by bacteria; is the least severe; and it usually resolves itself.

Meningitis is transmitted by direct contact with nose and throat fluids, usually through kissing, coughing, sneezing, or sharing drinks, cigarettes, or food. Children and young adults are at the highest risk for meningococcal disease. A vaccine is available that can prevent some, but not all, cases of meningitis. Antibiotics have decreased the rate of deaths caused by meningitis, so early diagnosis and treatment of meningococcal disease is important. People who have suffered from meningitis and have recovered can have permanent hearing loss, kidney failure, or brain injury.

Viral meningitis is most commonly spread through direct contact of a noninfected person with the respiratory secretions (e.g., saliva, sputum, or nasal mucus) of an infected person. Maintaining good personal hygiene helps to reduce a person's risk of becoming infected with viral meningitis. The most effective means of prevention is for people to wash their hands thoroughly and often, as well as to clean contaminated surfaces with soap and hot water, and then disinfect such surfaces with a solution of chlorine-containing bleach made by mixing approximately ¼ cup of bleach with 1 gallon of water.

Tuberculosis

Tuberculosis (TB) is a communicable disease spread through airborne respiratory secretions (droplets), usually from coughing or sneezing. It is possible for TB bacteria to remain dormant in the human body for many years before causing active disease. People who have TB can be treated and cured with antibiotics; however, if TB patients do not take their medication as prescribed, the bacteria could become resistant to the medication and become a form of TB called multi-drug resistant TB.
(Source: www.cdc.gov/tb/)

People at the highest risk for TB are those over age 65, those with weakened immune systems, and those who were born in countries that have a high rate of TB. Currently, about one-third of the world's population is affected by TB, which continues to spread globally, resulting in approximately 8 million new cases and an estimated 2 million deaths each year. Measures used to prevent the spread of TB include vaccination, as well as the testing and treating of people who are in regular contact with infected people.

Sexually Transmitted Diseases (also known as Sexually Transmitted Infections (STIs))

Sexually transmitted diseases (STDs) are a major public health concern in all countries. The WHO has indicated that, in developing countries, STDs and related complications are among the top five disease categories for which adults seek medical care. In these countries, STDs, excluding HIV, are second only to child-bearing factors as the cause of diseases and death for women of childbearing age. In the United States, approximately one out of four young people currently have or have had an STD. African Americans and Hispanics have higher rates of STDs than do whites.

Typically, women suffer more serious symptoms and complications from STDs than men do, including pelvic inflammatory disease, infertility, ectopic pregnancies, chronic pelvic pain, and cervical cancer. In addition, the presence of an untreated STD can increase the risk and transmission of HIV exponentially.

Factors that contribute to the rapid spread of STDs include the following:

- mild or no symptoms, which results in people not getting treatment and unknowingly spreading diseases to others;
- the reluctance of Americans to discuss sexual behavior;
- poverty and marginalization of people in high-risk behavior groups (e.g., sex workers, adolescents, prisoners, and migrant workers)
- alcohol and drug abuse,
- the exchange of sex for drugs,
- anonymous and multiple sex partners,
- not using condoms, and
- a lack of belief in medical treatment.

If they are diagnosed early on, many bacterial STDs can be treated and cured fairly easily. Thus, it is important that public health agencies expand access to testing and treatment facilities for STDs, and also to educate people about safe sex and risk reduction, especially for young people, who have disproportionately high rates of STDs.

Hepatitis

Hepatitis A, B, and C are the most common types of **hepatitis**, which is a viral disease that affects the liver. There are vaccines to prevent hepatitis A and B, but there are none for hepatitis C.

Hepatitis A (HAV)

- HAV is found in the feces of people infected with the virus. This disease can cause people to become very ill, but often, it can be cured within six months. Good personal hygiene, especially frequent and careful hand washing, is the best prevention from contracting HAV.
- HAV often is found in parts of the world that have poor sanitation and sewage practices. In these areas, people become infected with HAV by eating or drinking contaminated food or water.
- HAV is classified as a sexually transmitted disease because it can be spread through sexual contact. Thus, the use of condoms or dental dams can help to prevent the risk of infection.

Symptoms of HAV include the following:

- a short, mild, flu-like illness,
- nausea, vomiting, and diarrhea,
- loss of appetite,
- weight loss,
- jaundice (yellowing of the skin and the whites of the eyes; darker yellow urine and pale feces),
- itchy skin, and
- abdominal pain.

Hepatitis B (HBV)

- HBV is transmitted from person to person through blood or other bodily fluids. It can also be passed from an infected pregnant woman to her fetus.
- HBV is more serious than HAV and can be a lifelong infection. It can cause cirrhosis of the liver, liver cancer, liver failure, and death.
- It is estimated that it is between 50 to 100 times more infectious than HIV is.
- Many people who become infected with HBV experience mild symptoms or no symptoms at all; however, they are still carriers of the virus and can pass it on to others.
- Most adults who have been infected with HBV and are treated fully recover and develop life-long immunity.

HBV can be spread in the following ways:

- having unprotected sex with an infected person,
- sharing contaminated needles and other devices for drug use,
- using non-sterilized equipment for tattooing, acupuncture, or body piercing,
- passing from an infected mother to her baby during delivery. (Immunization of the baby at birth prevents the transmission of HBV.), and
- through a blood transfusion in a country where blood is not screened for HBV. (In the United States, all blood to be used for transfusions is tested.)

Hepatitis B can cause the following complications:

- chronic hepatitis,
- cirrhosis of the liver, and
- liver cancer.

Hepatitis C (HCV)

- HCV causes inflammation of the liver. It is transferred primarily through blood, and it is a more serious disease than either hepatitis A or B.

HCV can be spread in the following ways:

- sharing contaminated needles and other devices for drug use, including devices used to snort cocaine, as these can be contaminated with blood from a user's nose
- using non-sterilized equipment for tattooing, acupuncture, or body piercing,
- exposure to blood (from menstruation, genital sores, or cuts) during unprotected sex with an infected person,
- through a blood transfusion in a country where blood is not screened for HVC

Symptoms of HCV may include the following:

- a short, mild, flu-like illness,
- nausea and vomiting,
- diarrhea,
- loss of appetite,
- weight loss,
- jaundice (the yellowing of skin and the whites of the eyes, darker yellow urine, and pale feces), and
- itchy skin.

For an estimated 20% of people who become infected with HCV, their bodies will eliminate the virus within six months, while the other 80% will develop a chronic hepatitis C infection.

Hepatitis C can cause the following complications:

- chronic hepatitis,
- cirrhosis of the liver, and
- liver cancer.

Examples of Noncommunicable Diseases

Diabetes

Diabetes is actually two diseases that are characterized by high levels of blood glucose that result from defects in insulin production, insulin action, or both. Although diabetes can lead to severe complications and premature death, people who have the disease can take measures to control it, thereby lowering their risk for complications. Currently one of the leading causes of death and disability in the United States diabetes is also the fastest growing chronic disease in U.S. history. As many as 2,000 people are diagnosed with diabetes every day in the United States. Approximately 73% of people who have diabetes also have high blood pressure, and smoking doubles the risk for heart disease in those with diabetes.

- **Type 1 Diabetes** (formerly called juvenile diabetes) occurs when the body's own immune system attacks and destroys its insulin-producing beta cells in the pancreas. People with type 1 diabetes need to have insulin delivered by injections or with a pump. Some symptoms of type 1 diabetes include increased thirst and urination, constant hunger, weight loss, blurred vision, and fatigue. When a person who has type 1 diabetes is not diagnosed and treated, he or she can lapse into a life-threatening coma. Approximately 5% to 10% of all diagnosed cases of diabetes are type 1 diabetes.

- **Type 2 Diabetes** (formerly called adult-onset diabetes) results when the body does not make enough insulin or cannot effectively use the insulin that it does make. Type 2 diabetes is a lifestyle disease, usually caused by poor eating habits and a sedentary lifestyle. At one time, type 2 diabetes typically developed in adults over age 40; however, it is now becoming much more common in much younger people, including adolescents and even children. Some symptoms of type 2 diabetes include unusual thirst, frequent urination (especially at night), fatigue, blurred vision, frequent infections, and slow healing of wounds. Approximately 90% to 95% of all diagnosed cases of diabetes are type 2 diabetes.

Risk factors of type 2 diabetes:

- a family history of diabetes,
- being African Americans, Native American, or Hispanic (On average, African Americans are 1.8 times more likely to have diabetes as are non-Hispanic whites of similar age.),
- being overweight or obese,
- having had diabetes while pregnant (gestational diabetes),
- having high blood pressure,
- having abnormal cholesterol (lipid) levels, and
- not getting enough physical activity.

Overweight adults and children can sometimes prevent or delay type 2 diabetes. Those who already have diabetes can manage it by eating healthful foods, being physically active, and testing their blood glucose levels. The risk of developing complications from diabetes can be reduced or delayed significantly by keeping blood glucose (blood sugar), blood pressure, and cholesterol levels (called the ABCs of diabetes) within the target range. Gestational diabetes is high blood sugar that starts or is first diagnosed during pregnancy.

Risk factors for gestational diabetes include:

- African or Hispanic ancestry
- Being older than 25 when pregnant
- Family history of diabetes
- Giving birth to a previous baby that weighed more than 9 pounds
- Obesity
- Recurrent infections
- Unexplained miscarriage or death of a newborn.

There is a slightly increased risk of the baby dying when the mother has untreated gestational diabetes. Controlling blood sugar levels reduces this risk.

The National Diabetes Education Program (NDEP) recommends the following targets for reducing risk of heart disease and stroke:

Hemoglobin A1C (Blood Glucose over 8–12 weeks): Less than 6 percent

Blood Pressure: Less than 130/80 mmHg

Cholesterol: Less than 200 mg/dl

Triglycerides: Below 150

The following can help a person with type 2 diabetes manage the disease:

- Lose 5% to 7% percent of his or her body weight (i.e., 10 to 15 pounds for a person who weighs 200 pounds).
- Engage in physical activity for thirty minutes a day, five days a week.
- Make more healthful food choices, and limit the amount of calories and fat in his or her diet.

Cardiovascular Disease

The heart is a muscle and needs a constant supply of oxygen and nutrients that are carried to it by the blood.

Heart disease occurs when the normal functioning of the heart is impaired.

One form of heart disease is **atherosclerosis,** which is a thickening of the coronary arteries that narrows the space through which blood can flow, sometimes completely cutting off the supply of oxygen and nutrients to the heart.

Angina is a condition in which not enough oxygen-carrying blood reaches the heart, and the heart often responds with pain. A **heart attack** occurs when the blood supply to the heart is cut off completely. The part of the heart that does not receive oxygen begins to die, and some of the heart muscle may be permanently damaged.

Atherosclerosis usually is the result of a person having too high a level of cholesterol.

Cholesterol is a fatlike substance that circulates in the blood. It can build up on the walls of the arteries, thereby narrowing the arteries and slowing or blocking the flow of blood. Animal products contain the highest amount of dietary cholesterol. Cholesterol is also manufactured by the liver.

High blood cholesterol, high blood pressure, and smoking all contribute to heart disease. On average, each of these factors doubles a person's risk of developing heart disease. Thus, a person who has all three risk factors is about eight times more likely to develop heart disease than is a person who has none of these risk factors. Being overweight or obese increases the likelihood of a person developing high blood cholesterol and high blood pressure, and leading a sedentary lifestyle increases the risk of heart attack.

The best preventive measures to control the risk factors for developing heart disease include the following:

- regular exercise,
- good nutrition, and
- and not smoking.

Risk factors that you can control:

- Avoid tobacco.
- Cut down on saturated fats and cholesterol.
- Maintain a healthful weight.
- Maintain healthful dietary habits.
- Exercise regularly.
- Control diabetes.
- Control high blood pressure.
- Manage stress.

Risk factors that you cannot control:

- Heredity
- Age
- Gender
- Race

Cancer

Cancer is a group of diseases in which abnormal cells divide uncontrollably and are able to invade other tissues. When the genetic material (DNA) of a cell becomes damaged or changes, mutations can result and adversely affect normal cell growth and division. As a result, cells do not die when they should, and new cells form when the body does not need them. The extra cells can form a mass of tissue called a **tumor.**

There are more than 100 different known types of cancer. Most types of cancer are named for the organ or type of cell in which they start; for example, cancer that begins in the pancreas is called pancreatic cancer, and cancer that begins in basal cells of the skin is called basal cell carcinoma.

(Source: http://www.cancer.gov/cancertopics/types/pancreatic)

Cancer can cause many different symptoms, including the following:

- a thickening or lump in the breast or any other part of the body
- the development of a new mole or a change in an existing mole
- a sore that does not heal
- hoarseness or a cough that does not go away
- changes in bowel or bladder habits
- discomfort after eating
- difficulty swallowing
- weight gain or loss with no known reason
- unusual bleeding or discharges
- fatigue

Usually, these symptoms are not a result of cancer. They might be caused by other health problems or by a benign tumor. Only a doctor or doctors can make a diagnosis. A person who has any of these symptoms or any other changes in health should see a doctor so that he or she can diagnose and treat any health problems as early as possible.

(Source: http://www.cancer.gov/cancertopics/factsheet/Sites-Types/general)

Risk factors for cancer that you can control:

1. **Tobacco**

Using tobacco products or regularly being around tobacco smoke (environmental or secondhand smoke) increases the risk of cancer. The use of tobacco is the most preventable cause of death. More than 180,000 Americans die every year from tobacco-related cancer.

Anyone who uses tobacco should quit. Even those who have used tobacco for many years or even decades lower their risk of developing cancer by quitting.

2. **Sunlight**

Ultraviolet (UV) radiation comes from the sun, sunlamps, and tanning booths. UV radiation causes premature aging of the skin and skin damage, which can lead to skin cancer.

According to the American Cancer Society, most of the more than 1 million cases of non-melanoma skin cancer diagnosed each year in the United States are considered to be sun-related. Melanoma, the most serious type of skin cancer, accounted for about 60,000 cases of skin cancer in 2007, and for most (about 8,000) of the approximately 11,000 deaths caused by skin cancer each year. An estimated one in five Americans will develop skin cancer in their lifetimes.

The number of cases of skin cancer has been rising over the years. Many doctors believe that this is a result of the popularity of tanning beds as well as to people spending more time in the sun without properly using sunscreen.

Risk factors for skin cancer:

- unprotected and/or excessive exposure to ultraviolet (UV) radiation;
- a fair complexion;
- occupational exposures to coal tar, pitch, creosote, arsenic compounds, or radium;
- family history;
- multiple or a typical moles; and
- severe sunburns as a child.

Signs and symptoms of skin cancer:

- any changes on the skin, especially in the size, shape or color of a mole or other darkly pigmented growth or patch, or a new growth
- scaliness, oozing, bleeding, or changes in the appearance of a bump or nodule
- the spread of pigmentation beyond a previous border, such as dark coloring that spreads beyond the edges of a mole or birthmark
- sensations in the skin such as itchiness, tenderness, and pain

(Source: http://www.cancer.gov/cancertopics/types/skin)

Adequate protection from the sun is the best means of lowering the risk of non-melanoma skin cancer.

Preventive measures for avoiding skin cancer include the following:

- avoid being in direct sunlight between 10 A.M. and 4 P.M.
- take shelter under shade, especially in the middle of the day, when the sun's rays are strongest.
- cover as much skin as possible with protective clothing to guard against exposure when you are out in the sun.
- use sunscreen with a sun protection factor (SPF) of 15 or higher. Apply sunscreen liberally to skin and reapply after swimming or perspiring. Use sunscreen even on hazy or overcast days, as the sun's UV rays penetrate clouds.
- cover your head with a wide-brimmed hat to shade your face, ears, and neck.
- wear sunglasses with 99% to 100% UV absorption.
- avoid tanning beds and sun lamps.

3. **Certain Chemicals and Other Substances**

People who work in certain jobs (such as painters, construction workers, and those who work in the chemical industry) have an increased risk for cancer. Studies have shown that prolonged exposure to asbestos, benzene, benzidine, cadmium, nickel, vinyl chloride, and other chemicals in workplaces may cause certain types of cancers.

Workers in these jobs should be aware of the substances with which they are working and wear protective clothing, including gloves, and in some cases, face masks and goggles.

4. **Some Viruses and Bacteria**

Being infected with certain viruses or bacteria, such as the following, may increase the risk of developing cancer:

- **Human papillomaviruses (HPV):** HPV infection is the main cause of cervical cancer.
- **Hepatitis B and hepatitis C viruses:** Liver cancer can develop after many years of hepatitis B or hepatitis C infection.
- **Human T-cell leukemia/lymphoma virus (HTLV-1):** Infection with HTLV-1 increases 'the risk of the development of lymphoma and leukemia.
- **Human immunodeficiency virus (HIV):** HIV is the virus that causes AIDS. Those who have HIV are at increased risk for some cancers, such as lymphoma and a rare cancer called Kaposi's sarcoma.
- **Epstein-Barr virus (EBV):** Infection with EBV has been associated with an increased risk of lymphoma.
- **Human herpes virus 8 (HHV8):** An HHV8 infection is a risk factor for Kaposi's sarcoma.
- **Helicobacter pylori:** This bacterium can stomach cancer and lymphoma in the stomach lining, as well as stomach ulcers.

5. **Certain Hormones**

Some women are prescribed certain hormones, such as estrogen alone or estrogen along with progestin, to help control symptoms of menopause, including hot flashes, vaginal dryness, and thinning bones. However, studies have shows that menopausal hormone therapy can cause serious side effects and may increase the risk of breast cancer, heart attack, stroke, and blood clots.

6. **Alcohol**

A person who has more than two alcoholic drinks every day over a long period of time may have increased chances of developing several types of cancer, including mouth, throat, esophagus, larynx, liver, and breast cancers. The chances increase with increased amounts of alcohol, for most of these cancers, the risk also increased for a drinker who uses tobacco.

7. **Poor Diet, Lack of Physical Activity, and Being Overweight**

A poor diet, an inadequate amount of physical activity, and being overweight or obese may place people at increased risks for several different types of cancer. For example, studies suggest that people who have high-fat diets have a greater chance of developing cancer of the colon, uterus, and prostate. Leading a sedentary lifestyle and being overweight are risk factors for breast, colon, esophagus, kidney, and uterine cancers.
(Source: http://www.cancer.gov/cancertopics/energybalance)

The World's Healthiest People

The World's Top 10 Countries with the Healthiest People

1. Japan
2. Switzerland
3. San Marino
4. Sweden
5. Australia
6. France

7. Monaco
8. Iceland
9. Austria
10. Italy

Japan has the healthiest (and some of the oldest) people in the world. There, the average life expectancy is 86 years of age for women and 79 years of age for men, A healthful diet that is rich in seaweed and fish and low in fat, as well as government-sponsored exercise programs, contribute to the longevity of the Japanese people. The healthiest people on Earth live in Okinawa, Japan. It has the highest number of people who are 100 years or older per capita of any area or country in the world–more than three times the number for Americans. Compared with the high incidence of heart disease in the United States, Okinawans have few incidences of heart disease. They also have 80% less cases of breast and prostate cancer, 50% less cases of colon and ovarian cancer, and 40% fewer hip fractures.

Factors for longevity in Okinawans:

1. Okinawans live calm, peaceful lives, with little stress and positive, optimistic attitudes.
2. They tend to form strong social relationships. Okinawans often get together with friends and family to offer support to one another. Many studies have shown that people who have several good relationships with others and that lead active, positive social lives are healthier than those who don't.
3. Okinawans have a healthful, wholesome diet. The traditional Okinawa diet consists mainly of fish that is rich with protein and omega-3 oils and plant foods that have high levels of vitamins, minerals, and phytonutrients. In addition, Okinawans generally do not overeat, eating between 500 and 1,000 fewer calories per day than does an average American.
4. Most Okinawans get plenty of exercise by walking a lot and practicing traditional martial arts, such as tai chi.
5. Few Okinawans, especially those who are older, smoke tobacco or drink alcohol.

Other countries that have high rates of longevity include Germany, Switzerland, Australia, Denmark, Canada, Austria, and the Netherlands. These countries have very high-quality drinking water, sanitation, and nutritional levels. Iceland and Sweden have some of the lowest levels of air pollution, infant mortality rates, and rates of tuberculosis. They also share the highest life expectancies for men.

(Source: http://www.forbes.com/forbes/2009/0921/opinions-health-life-expectancy-on-my-mind.html)

Factors for longevity in the countries with the world's healthiest people:

- **These countries all share one thing in common: a nationalized health care system.**
- **Sweden** has high rates of cancer survival and excellent health care for children. The Swedish approach to health care is holistic, promoting health as including lifestyle as well as medical care. One example of this approach is providing well-lit public places to promote evening walks.
- **Italy** has a tradition of using fresh, unprocessed foods and on home cooking rather than buying prepared, packaged foods.
- **Iceland** has world's healthiest infants, with only two deaths before the age of 5 for every 1,000 births. Iceland places a heavy emphasis on health care, offering extensive prenatal and post-birth health care for mothers and children. In addition, parents are guaranteed three months of paid professional leave for the birth of every child.
- **Cuba** offers some of the best health care in the world because it focuses on early detection and prevention of diseases, despite its shortage of some medical equipment.
- **Finland** had the highest death rate from heart disease among men thirty years ago. Thus, the government began to promote healthful lifestyles, including greater consumption of fruits and vegetables. Finland now has a low rate of heart disease, as well as one of the lowest infant mortality rates in the world.
- **France** has a low rate of heart disease, despite the high fat content of French food. This is partly because the French tend to eat small portions of food, eat their meals slowly, and use fresh, wholesome ingredients in cooking and baking.

References

American Cancer Society, *Skin Cancer Facts 2009,* www.acs.org.

Adler, N.E., & Newman, K., "Socioeconomic disparities in health: pathways and policies; inequality in education, income, and occupation exacerbates the gaps between the health 'haves' and 'have-nots,'" *Health Affairs,* 21(2) (2002;): 60–76.

Clayton, David, and Michel Hills, *Statistical Models in Epidemiology.* Oxford: Oxford University Press, 1993.

Collins J., Robin L., Wooley, S., Fenley, D., Hunt, P., Taylor, J., Haber, D., & Kolbe L., "Programs that work: CDC's guide to effective programs that reduce health-risk behavior of youth," *Journal of School Health;* 72 (2002): 93–99.

Connell, J.P., Halpern-Felsher, B.L., Clifford E., et al., "Hanging in there: Behvaioral, psychological and contextual factors affecting whether African-American adolescents stay in school," *Journal of Adolescent Research* 10 (1995): 41–63.

Christenson, L.J., "Incidence of basal cell and squamous cell carcinomas in a population younger than 40 years," *Journal of the American Medical Association,* vol. 294, No. 6: (2006): 681–690.

Diabetes Education Program, www.ndep.nih.gov.

Ensminger, M.E., Lamkin, R.P., $ Jacobson, N., "School leaving: A longitudinal perspective including neighborhood effects." *Child Development* 67 (1996): 2400–2416.

Fisher, C., Hunt, P., Kann, L., Kolbe, L., Patterson, B., & Wechsler, H,. "Building a healthier future through school health programs, *US CDC,* February 2005. Available at http://www.cdc.gov/nccdphp/promising_practices/school_health/index.htm

H. Krauss, A. Weber, M. Appel, B. Enders, A. v. Graevenitz, H. D. Isenberg, H. G. Schiefer, W. Slenczka, & H. Zahner-Zoonoses, *Infectious Diseases Transmissible from Animals to Humans,* 3rd ed.,. (Washington, D.C.: American Society for Microbiology,Press, 2003.

http://en.wikipedia.org/wiki/Epidemiology Centers for Disease Control and Prevention. "Unrealized prevention opportunities: Reducing the health and economic burden of chronic disease," National Center for Chronic Disease Prevention and Health Promotion, *Chronic Disease Prevention,* November 1998.

Institute of Medicine. *Dietary Reference Intakes: Energy, Carbohydrate, Fiber, Fat, Fatty Acids, Cholesterol, Protein, and Amino Acids* (Washington, D.C.: National Academy Press, 2002). (See chapter 12.)

Kenneth J. Ryan & C. George Ray, *Sherris Medical Microbiology,* 4th ed. (McGraw Hill Medical Publishing: 2004).

Key, T.J., Allen, N.E., Spencer, E.A., "The effect of diet on risk of cancer," Lancet. 2002 Sep 14; 360 (9336):861–8.

Kirby, D., "The impact of schools and school programs upon adolescent sexual behavior," *Journal of Sex Research* 39 (2002): 27–33.

Last, J.M., *A Dictionary of Epidemiology*, 4th ed. (Oxford: Oxford University Press, 2001).

Link, B.G. & Phelan, J., "Social conditions as fundamental causes of disease," *Journal of Health and Social Behavior;* extra issue (1995); 80–94.

McGraw-Hill Encyclopedia of Science and Technology, "Infectious disease," The McGraw-Hill Medical Publishing, 2005.

Molla, M.T., Madans, J.H., Wagener, D.K., "Differentials in adult mortality and activity limitation by years of education in the United States at the end of the 1990s," *Population and Development Review* 30 (2004): 625–646.

Morabia, Alfredo, ed., *A History of Epidemiologic Methods and Concepts:. Part I.* Basel: Birkhauser Verlag, 2004.

Morone, J.A., Kilbreth, E., & Langwell, K.M., "Back to school: A heath care strategy for youth," *Health Affairs* 20 (2001): 122–36.

Pastor, P.N., D.M. Makuc, C. Reuben, H. Xia, et al., *Chartbook on Trends in the Health of Americans, Health, United States, 2002* (Hyattsville, MD: National Center for Health Statistics, 2002. (Online trend data available at http://www.cdc.gov/nchs/products/pubs/pubd/hus/02hustop.htm)

Phillips, C.V. & Goodman, K.J., "The missed lessons of Sir Austin Bradford Hill," *Epidemiologic Perspectives and Innovations*, 1 (2004): 3.

Smith, S.S., "Health in the U.S. tied to income and education." *U.S. Department of Health and Human Services Public Health Reports* (1998), 113: 557.

Smolinski, M.S., Hamburg, M.A., Lederberg, J., eds., *Microbial Threats to Health: Emergence, Detection, and Response.* Washington, D.C.: The National Academics Press, 2003.

Stein, C.J., & Colditz, G.A., "The epidemic of obesity," *Journal of Clinical Endocrinology and Metabolism* 89(6) (2004): 2522–2525.

Stringer, S., "Failing grade: Health education in NYC schools," Report by NY State Assembly Member Scott Stringer, June 2003.

Symons C.W., Cinelli B., James, T.C., & Groff, P., "Bridging student health risks and academic achievement through comprehensive school health programs," *Journal of School Health* 67 (1997): 220–227.

Szklo, M.M. & Nieto, F.J., *Epidemiology: Beyond the Basics,* Aspen: Aspen Publishers, Inc., 2002.

United Nations, *Demographic Yearbook 1999,* New York: United Nations, 2001, 479–506.

U.S. Department of Health and Human Services, National Institute of Health, "National Diabetes Statistics Fact Sheet: General Information and National Estimates on Diabetes in the United States, 2005."

Wagner, E.H., Austin, B.T., Davis, C, Hindmarsh, M, Schaefer J, & Bonomi A., "Improving chronic illness care: translating evidence into action," *Health Affairs* 20(6) (2001): 64–77

www.cancer.org.

Chapter

4

HEALTH DISPARITIES

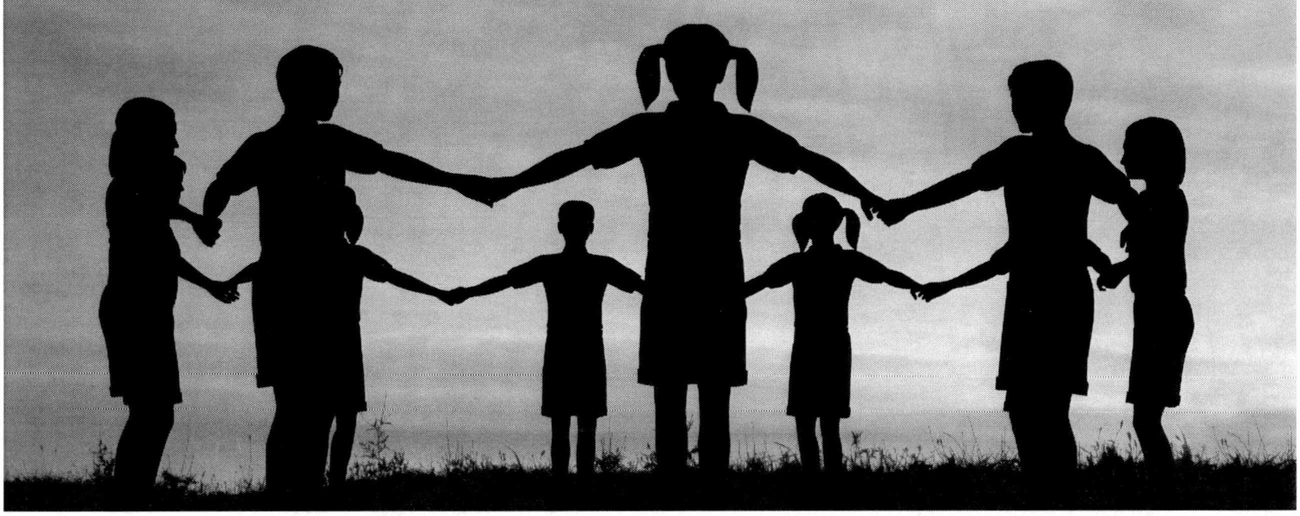

"The greatest single challenge facing our globalized world is to combat and eradicate its disparities."

—Nelson Mandela

Cultural, ethnic, and racial diversity remains one of the strengths of the United States as our population continues to grow. However, there are significant disparities in health between various minorities and the general population. Inequalities in health are based upon observable differences, or disparities, in the health of different populations.

Health disparities are differences in the occurrences, prevalence, mortality, and burden of diseases, as well as other detrimental health conditions, which exist among specific population groups. Such disparities occur when a group, whether it be a gender, race, ethnicity, or community, has a higher predisposition for disease or illness than does the larger population to which it belongs.

When there is a significant difference in the overall rate of incidences and prevalence of disease, morbidity, mortality, or survival rates in a specific part of a population in comparison with the health status of the general population, a **health disparity population** exists.

An example of a health disparity is the **infant mortality rate,** which is the number of children who die before they reach age 1 divided by the number of live births that year. The infant mortality rate is the most significant measure of the well-being of infants in any given population.

Factors that influence an infant mortality rate include the following:

- the health of the mother,
- the quality of and access to medical care,
- socioeconomic conditions,
- environmental conditions, and
- public health practices.

In the United States, the infant mortality rate of whites is 5.9 per 1,000, whereas the rate for African-Americans is 13.9 per 1,000. The difference between the two rates clearly indicates that there are health disparities between these two groups in the overall population.

Contributors to health disparities include the following:

- not having health insurance or having inadequate health insurance,
- racism and other "isms" that decrease opportunities or cause discrimination,
- lack of transportation,
- lifestyle behaviors,
- cultural influences, customs, and beliefs,
- a poor diet,
- a lack of exercise,
- obesity or being overweight,
- unsafe sexual behaviors,
- stress,
- mental health issues,
- systemic barriers,
- access to health care,
- poverty, and
- environmental factors.

Why Is Diversity Significant?

By the year 2050, nearly half of the U.S. population will be composed of racial minorities. As we move into the future, health-care systems are and will continue to deal with a much more diverse and less healthy population. Health disparities in the United States are not new phenomena; they have existed throughout our history. Health disparities for ethnic and racial minorities continue to be a community problem, with not nearly enough progress having been made to eliminate them.

The most common health disparities known to exist in the United States relate to heart disease, cancer, diabetes, accidental injuries, and HIV/AIDS. According to former Surgeon General David Satcher, the mortality rate for heart disease is more than 40% higher for African Americans than for whites. The mortality rate for all types of cancer is 30% higher for African Americans than it is for whites, with African American women experiencing higher mortality rates from breast cancer, despite an increase in screening for this group. The incidence of prostate cancer for African American men is more than double that of white men. For African Americans, the rate of HIV/AIDS is more than seven times the rate for whites, and, specifically for African American women, the incidence of HIV is as much as 20 times higher than it is for white women. As for homicide, the rate is six times higher for African Americans than it is for whites.

*(Source: www.cdc.gov/**hiv**/pubs/facts/**women**.htm)*

Causes of death that are highest among minorities in United States include the following:

- **Infant mortality:** the highest predictor of overall health in a population, this is often a result of a lack of access to good prenatal care;
- **Cancer:** the rate of deaths is high because of a lack of screening;
- **Cardiovascular disease and stroke:** both are caused by hypertension, obesity, poor diet; and unhealthful lifestyle behaviors;

- **Diabetes type 2:** is a result of a poor diet, obesity, and a sedentary lifestyle;
- **Homicide and accidents:** these often result from poverty and negative social and/or living conditions;
- **Chemical dependence:** is often a result of a low level of education and low income.

Health disparities in the United States are most common among the four main ethnic or racial groups in this country: African Americans, Hispanics, Asian/Pacific Islanders, and Native Americans. Historically, these groups, as well as immigrants, the poor, and the mentally challenged, have not received the level of health care that the general population has, which is reflected by their high morbidity and mortality rates.

African Americans

African Americans make up an estimated 13% (36 million people), or less than one-sixth, of the U.S. population. However, this group experiences a disproportionate amount of diseases, injuries, death, and disabilities resulting from a variety of medical conditions as compared with other racial or ethnic groups and with the general population. Disparities in the socioeconomic status of African Americans as compared with whites include higher unemployment and underemployment, lower levels of education, discrimination, and more poverty among African Americans. All of these factors contribute significantly to disparities in their health status.

Health disparities between African Americans and whites include the following:

- African Americans have higher rates of morbidity and mortality for many chronic diseases that are associated with a poor diet and obesity.
- The mortality rate for cancer of African-American men is 1.4 times higher than it is for white men, and for African-American women, that rate is 1.2 times higher than it is for white women.
- The life expectancy of African Americans is lower than it is for whites.
- Sickle-cell anemia is another disease that disproportionately afflicts African Americans. An estimated 1 out of 12 African Americans is born with the sickle cell trait, and about 1 out of 375 is born with sickle cell anemia.

Sickle cell anemia is a disease in which the body manufactures sickle-shaped (or crescent-shaped) red blood cells instead of the normally C-shaped red blood cells. An abnormal hemoglobin level causes these cells to have their sickle shape, which prevents them from moving easily through the blood vessels. Instead of being smooth and able to glide easily, sickle cells are stiff and sticky, and they are prone to clumping and getting stuck in the blood vessels. When this happens, the clumps of sickle cells block the flow of blood in the blood vessels that lead to the limbs and internal organs. Blood vessels that are blocked can cause pain, severe infections, and organ damage. Sickle cell anemia is an inherited, lifelong disease. People who have the disease are born with it. They inherit two copies of the sickle cell gene—one from each parent. (Source: NHLBI.gov)

Hispanics

In 2008, Hispanics made up account 15.4% of the population of the United States, making them the largest minority group in the country. This percentage is expected to continue to grow.

Health disparities between Hispanics and non-Hispanic whites include the following:

- Mortality rates for accidents, homicide, and HIV/AIDS are higher for Americans of Hispanic origin than they are for non-Hispanic whites.
- Not only do Hispanics have higher mortality rates for diabetes than do non-Hispanic whites, but they are also twice as likely to die from this disease.
- Hispanics have higher rates of hypertension and obesity than do non-Hispanic whites.

For socioeconomic reasons, Hispanics as a group lag behind the general population in their levels of education. Both low levels of education and poverty contribute to the poorer health status of Hispanics as a group. In some cases, the immigration status of Hispanics leaves them with no access to health insurance and little access to health care.

Acculturation is the process by which immigrants adopt the attitudes, values, customs, beliefs and behaviors of the culture in their new country. The **Hispanic Paradox** is a theory that states that immigrants of Hispanic origin are healthier before they come to the United States and then go on to acculturate and take up unhealthful habits that are common in this country.

Greater acculturation is associated with the following:

- an increased rate of infant mortality and low birth weight,
- overall cancer rates,
- high blood pressure,
- adolescent pregnancies,
- smoking, alcohol consumption, and illicit drug use,
- decreased consumption of fiber
- depression

Asian/Pacific Islanders

While Asian/Pacific Islanders are one of the healthiest population groups, they still experience some health disparities.

Health disparities between Asian/Pacific Islanders and other groups include the following:

- The mortality rate of Vietnamese women with cervical cancer is five times higher than that of white women.
- The incidences of newly diagnosed cases of hepatitis and tuberculosis are higher for Asian/Pacific Islanders than they are for the general population.
- The incidence of tuberculosis (TB) for Asian/Pacific Islanders is nearly five times higher than that of the total population.
- Asians have a greater risk of contracting hepatitis B, and more Asian people are infected with hepatitis B than are non-Asians. In most cases, Asians become infected with the hepatitis B virus when they are infants or young children. This occurs when infected mothers unknowingly pass on the virus to their babies at birth or when infants or young children are exposed to blood from another infected person with whom they live in close contact. When these children become adults, their immune systems can usually rid their bodies of the virus, and they usually recover.

Despite certain health disparities, the infant mortality rate of Asian/Pacific Islanders is the lowest of any minority in the United States. This is a result of higher levels of education and better prenatal care than those of other minorities.

Native Americans

Native Americans account for only about 1% of the current population of the United States.

Health disparities between Native Americans and the general population include the following:

- Higher mortality rates, with a life expectancy of five years less than the national average;
- Higher rates of tuberculosis, chronic liver disease and cirrhosis of the liver, accidents, diabetes, pneumonia, influenza, suicide, and homicide;

- Alcohol abuse, which is a very serious problem in Native American communities as a result of physiological and social factors related to the historic changes in their cultures;
- Large families with lower levels of education and income than the general population, which causes a low health status

Like Asian/Pacific Islanders, however, Native Americans have very low rates of infant mortality.

Immigrants

A **refugee** is a person who flees from one country or area to seek shelter or protection from danger in another area or country. An **immigrant** is a person who migrates from one country into another to find a permanent residence. An **alien** has no citizenship in the country in which he or she is residing. Aliens must eventually return to their original countries. An **illegal alien** is a person who flees from their homeland into another country without proper authorization.

A recent report published by the New York City Department of Health and Mental Hygiene, entitled *The Health of Immigrants in New York City*, found that immigrants or foreign-born New Yorkers were less likely than native New Yorkers or other American-born New Yorkers to have health insurance and therefore were less likely to have their blood pressure and cholesterol levels checked; experienced greater psychological distress; were less likely to have colon cancer screenings, pap tests, and mammograms; were less likely to receive immunization shots for flu and pneumonia; had higher rates of intimate-partner murder of females; had higher rates of tuberculosis; and had a higher rate of births for teen mothers than did U.S. citizens. As Dr. Thomas Frieden, former Commissioner of the New York City Department of Health and Mental Hygiene, explained, within the immigrant population "each subgroup has a distinct health profile." For example, the report indicates that Russian immigrants tend to be heavier smokers; Panamanian- and Honduran immigrants are more likely to be obese; those from Ireland, Ghana, and Korea experience more episodes of binge drinking; and New Yorkers who were born in China had the highest mortality rate for liver cancer.

Although estimates vary significantly, some reports indicate that there are approximately 12 million people who are in the United States illegally. These illegal immigrants make up about 20% of the 46 million people who lack health insurance in the United States. In addition to those whose status is illegal and therefore cannot obtain health insurance, legal immigrants often have language barriers that prevent them from learning about health insurance coverage that might be available, understanding how to apply for health insurance, and even understanding how to maintain health insurance coverage. In addition, both language and cultural barriers present difficulties in communicating with doctors and other health-care providers, including clearly understanding medical instructions. Such difficulties in communication can lead to serious health problems. To help mitigate the problems in health care caused by language and cultural barriers, many states have mandated that state applications for health care programs be offered in multiple languages. In addition, some states are hiring outreach workers and medically trained interpreters to reduce the problems that arise from miscommunication.

The United States has two large health-care coverage programs available to immigrants: Medicaid and the State Children's Health Insurance Program (SCHIP).

- **Medicaid** is a government program that offers public assistance to people whose income and resources are insufficient to pay for health care.
- **SCHIP** is a program in which the federal government matches the funds of states to expand health insurance coverage to children.

Interventions to narrow the gap between immigrant and citizen health include the following:

- government and public health agencies working to lower the barriers to health insurance enrollment,
- reducing language and cultural barriers,
- alleviating immigrants' concerns about participation in government health programs, and
- providing education about the importance of obtaining health insurance and preventive health care.

Health Disparities between Genders

Gender inequalities are differences that exist between men and women that empower one group to the detriment of the other. As in the social and political arenas, gender inequalities also exist in health status and access to health care.

An estimated 500,000 women die each year from cardiovascular disease, a higher rate than for men; however, there is a gap in the awareness of the need to identify and treat women for heart disease.

A study conducted by the Society for Women's Health Research indicated that a mere 3% of the total U.S. health budget was allocated to the study of gender differences. In fact, up until 1990, most clinical trials excluded women because researchers were concerned about women's hormonal changes and how those changes might influence the results of the studies.

Examples of gender health disparities include the following:

- Health disparities because of gender might be related, in part, to the exclusion of women from many clinical trials because of researchers' concerns about reproductive or menstrual issues.
- The life expectancy for women in the United States is 79.8, a little more than five years longer than the life expectancy for men, which is 74.4. Although women tend to live longer than men, they don't necessarily enjoy a better quality of life. Women who are 100 years of age or older outnumber men by a ratio of eight to one.
- Mortality rates from cancer are higher for men than for women.
- Sleep apnea, a potentially serious disorder that causes breathing to stop and start repeatedly during sleep, is more common in men than in women.
- Four times as many men commit suicide as women.
- Men tend to have fewer infection-fighting T-cells than women do.
- Even allowing for differences in size, with equal amounts of consumption of alcohol, women have higher blood alcohol contents than men do.
- Women who smoke cigarettes are more likely to develop lung cancer than are men who smoke the same amount of cigarettes.
- Women are more likely than men are to suffer a second heart attack within one year of a first heart attack.
- The same drug can cause reactions and side effects that are different for women and men.
- Women are more likely than men are to acquire autoimmune diseases (diseases in which the body attacks its own tissues), such as lupus, rheumatoid arthritis, scleroderma, and multiple sclerosis.
- During unprotected intercourse with an infected partner, women are twice as likely as men are to contract a sexually transmitted disease, and 10 times more likely to contract HIV.
- Depression is two to three times more common in women than in men, partly because women's brains produce less of the hormone serotonin.
- After menopause, women lose more bone mass than men of similar age do.

Health Disparities in the Name of Science

"The United States government did something that was wrong—deeply, profoundly, morally wrong. It was an outrage to our commitment to integrity and equality for all our citizens . . . clearly racist."

—President Clinton's apology for the Tuskegee Syphilis Experiment to the eight remaining survivors, May 16, 1997

The Tuskegee Syphilis Experiment

Between 1932 and 1972, the U.S. Public Health Service (PHS) conducted an experiment on 399 African American men who were in the late stages of syphilis, a sexually transmitted disease (STD). Researchers never told these men what disease they had or informed them about how serious the disease is. The intention of the study was to discover how syphilis affects African Americans compared with whites. The theory was that syphilis made African Americans more susceptible to cardiovascular damage and that whites were more susceptible to neurological complications from the disease. The men participating in the study were simply told that they were being treated for "bad blood;" the doctors conducting the study had no intention of treating them for or curing them of syphilis. Even when penicillin became commercially available in 1945, it was intentionally withheld from the Tuskegee men participating in the experiment. By the end of the experiment, 28 of the men had died directly from syphilis, 100 had died from related complications, 40 of their wives had been infected, and 19 of their children had been born with congenital syphilis.

The Tuskegee experiment continued despite both the passage of the Henderson Act of 1943, a public health law that required testing and treatment for sexually transmitted diseases, and the World Health Organization's Declaration of Helsinki of 1964, which required "informed consent" from participants in experiments involving people.

Socioeconomic (SES) Disparities

"It is a crime to live in this rich nation and receive starvation wages."

—Dr. Martin Luther King Jr, in a speech to sanitation workers, 1968

The underlying causes of health disparities are disparities in socioeconomic status. **Socioeconomic status** is the place or position in society that a person or family has based on social, economic, and educational factors. More than 60 percent of people who have no health insurance have low incomes or are members of low-income families. For obvious reasons, people who do not have health insurance receive less medical care, including preventive care, screening, and treatment, than do people who are covered by health insurance. In addition, even when those with no health insurance coverage do receive medical care, it often is of a poorer quality than the care of those who have health insurance.

Low socioeconomic status is linked to a wide range of health problems, including the following:

- low birth weight;
- cardiovascular disease;
- hypertension;
- diabetes;
- cancer, with higher rates of mortality;
- arthritis;
- a sedentary lifestyle, which can lead to other health problems;
- inadequate consumption of fiber and fresh fruits and vegetables; and
- a high rate of tobacco use, which is the greatest behavioral risk for premature mortality.

Poverty creates conditions in which diseases frequently occur and spread, and are unlikely to be treated. More than a billion people throughout the world live on less than $1 per day.

Another health risk for people of low socioeconomic status is exposure to damaging substances in the environment. Such substances include lead, asbestos, carbon dioxide, and industrial wastes. These people are more likely than people of higher socioeconomic status to live and work in potentially harmful physical environments. In addition, poor neighborhoods often are located near highways, industrial areas, toxic waste sites, and other dangerous or unhealthful areas. As a result, people who live in such neighborhoods often have higher levels of lead in their blood, as well as higher rates of childhood asthma.

Did you know?

- An estimated 800,000 people in the United States are homeless on any given night.
- The gap between the rich and the poor has widened and continues to do so. Over the past two decades, the income gap has steadily risen, as the richest Americans, who own multiple homes, stocks, and many other assets and receive large tax breaks have become richer, while those at middle- and low-income levels have seen their buying power decrease.
- The assets of the top 1% richest Americans equals the combined wealth of the bottom 90%.
- In New York City, more than 800,000 children lived in poverty in 2009.
- Families with children make up 40% of homeless population.
- The average minimum-wage worker must work 89 hours per week to be able to afford a two-bedroom apartment.
- At the end of 2008, there were approximately 9,700 homeless families sleeping in municipal shelters in New York City, and about 3,300 living on the streets.
- Approximately 25 million Americans had to rely on soup kitchens, food banks, and shelters in 2006.
- Americans in need of food from charitable institutions included about 9 million children and 3 million senior citizens in 2006.

Hurricane Katrina

As millions of people watched with horror the aftermath of Hurricane Katrina in 2005 on television, many wondered how such a human disaster could have happened in the United States. Many people alternated between outrage and grief as they saw endless footage of the failure to materialize of the disaster relief services that we had assumed our government would provide. Appallingly, more than 1,000 citizens died because it took the government more than five days to distribute the necessary water, food, and medicine.

When one realizes who escaped the hurricane and its storm surge and who remained behind, it is impossible to ignore the shocking breadth of the gap between the rich and the poor. The reality is that poverty exists every day and in numerous places—it just isn't shown on TV as often as it was after Hurricane Katrina. For many of the more fortunate among us, the more than 37 million Americans living in poverty are unseen and unheard.

The Health Crisis Resulting from Hurricane Katrina

> *"What I'm hearing—which is sort of scary—is they all want to stay in Texas. Everyone is so overwhelmed by the hospitality. And so many of the people in the arena here, you know, were underprivileged anyway, so this—this is working very well for them.*
>
> —*former First Lady Barbara Bush, 2005*

According to the Centers for Disease Control and Prevention (CDC):

- One of most serious health concerns was the diseases and illnesses related to crowded conditions, such as diarrhea, colds, tuberculosis, and influenza.
- The mental health needs for hurricane survivors were also a major concern, as many people needed support and assistance dealing with their losses.

- The Environmental Protection Agency's test results for the floodwaters covering New Orleans found *E. coli* bacteria, as well as worrisome levels of lead. The CDC found that four deaths on the Gulf Coast resulted from infections caused by floodwater.
- One out of five survivors of the hurricane who requested Medicaid was rejected during the initial eligibility screenings because they did not fit Medicaid requirements.
- Seven neighborhoods in New Orleans had arsenic levels that were more than 100 times higher than levels that meet the Environmental Protection Agency's standards.
- There were 423 oil spills, natural gas spills, and other chemical spills off the coast of New Orleans.

Possible Solutions to Achieve Equality in Health

The quality of health-care services that are provided to minority groups and immigrants remains a major challenge in the United States.

Culturally Competent Health Care

Cultural competence is a set of skills, attitudes, and knowledge that enables people and organizations to work effectively with a diversity of ethnic, racial, and social groups. The existence of racial disparities in the incidences and prevalence of diseases, as well as health status, indicates that a system has not effectively responded to all the groups within a population.

The answers to the following questions can help determine whether or not a health care system in a community is culturally competent.

- Are staff members adequately trained to work with the diverse populations within the community that is being served?
- Can patients make a choice about whether they can see a provider from their own culture?
- Are beneficiaries from minority populations receiving critical and relevant interventions that address disparities?
- Are surveys reaching out to non-English speaking populations and trying to serve them?
- Do community outreach and education programs address disparities that are prevalent within the diverse populations of the community?
- Is there funding to support the institutionalization of cultural competence within the system or organization?
- Does the system or organization welcome and reach out to racial and ethnic groups in the target area?
- Is there diversity and representation of minority professionals and managers within the system or organization?

Solutions to End Health Disparities among Subpopulations

- To reduce many disparities in the health status of different groups of the American population, it is essential to address the issue of poverty.
- Universal health-care services would significantly improve the health of those in minority groups and would narrow the gap in the health status between minorities and the general population.
- People and communities must be empowered to pursue solutions to their own problems by acquiring the following:
  - **Social Power:** information, skills, and participation in social organizations,
  - **Political Power:** holding one's government accountable by voting and joining political organizations, and
  - **Psychological Power:** self-esteem, which leads to change.

- The promotion of wellness and healthful lifestyles is essential to the reduction and elimination of the unequal burden of disease mortality and morbidity that ethnic and racial groups currently endure. Because their social environment profoundly affects people's health, it is important to establish accessible exercise programs and to work towards decreasing violence in the neighborhoods of minorities.
- In addition to the social environment, the personal choices that people make, including interactions with family, friends, and members of the community are important factors to consider in attempting to eliminate disparities in the health status of ethnic and racial minority groups.
- Public officials should be held to high standards. When communities become actively involved in the political process in their communities, they can avert crises in political leadership.

  The following are ways in which people can become involved and empowered:

  - Vote.
  - Write or e-mail concerns and opinions to political representatives.
  - Organize letter-writing campaigns and enlist as many other people as possible.
  - Write letters to the editors of local newspapers.
  - Visit the Web site RESULTS.org, which contains many useful tools that can be adapted to help target politicians and media outlets.
  - Join existing networks, such as the Global Call to Action Against Poverty at http://www.whiteband.org/, which has national chapters in many countries.

Some questions to consider:

- What levels of poverty, hunger, and homelessness can we as a society tolerate, while claiming to be a compassionate country?
- What is the appropriate minimum wage, and how can people with low-paying jobs supplement their incomes?
- What new policy strategies can we develop to address discrimination based on ethnicity, race, and gender that leads to health disparities?
- How can our government provide all of its citizens with the basic human needs: food, shelter, health care, and wages that they can live on?
- How can our country move forward in providing equal opportunities to its most disadvantaged citizens?

Use your privileged, educated eyes to see the burdens of those who are less privileged and to help them. In whatever career you find yourself, become an agent of change to work towards ensuring that a fair and equal opportunity is available for *all!*

REFERENCES

Ayanian, J., Udvarhelyi, I., Gatsonis, C., Pashos, C., & Epstein, A., "Racial differences in the use of revascularization procedures after coronary angiography," *Journal of the American Medical Association* 269 (1993):642–646.

Association of American Medical Colleges. *Minority Graduates of U.S. Medical Schools: Trends, 1950–1998* (Washington, D.C.: Author, 2000).

Baldwin, D., "A model for describing low-income African American women's participation breast and cervical cancer early detection and screening," *Advances in Nursing Science* 19 (1996): 27–42.

Baldwin, D. & Nelms, T., "Difficult dialogues: Impact on nursing education curricula." *Journal of Professional Nursing* 9(6) (1993) 3343–3346.

Bartlett, D., "The new health care consumer," *Journal of Health Care Finance* 25 (1999):44–51.

Brown E.R., Pourat, N., Wallace, S.P, "Undocumented residents make up small share of California's uninsured population," (Los Angeles: UCLA Center for Health Policy Research, March 2007).

Byrne, M, "Uncovering racial bias in fundamental nursing textbooks: A critical hermeneutic analysis of the portrayal of African Americans," unpublished dissertation (Georgia State University: Atlanta, 2000).

Chen, M. S., & Hawks, B. L., "A debunking of the myth of healthy Asian Americans and Pacific Islanders," *American Journal of Health Promotion*, 9(4) (1995): 261–268.

Collins, K., Hall, A., & Neuhaus, C., *U.S. Minority health: A chartbook.* (New York: The Commonwealth Fund, 1999).

Cooper-Patrick, L., Gallo, J., Gonzales, J, Vu., H., Powe, N., Nelson, C., & Ford, D., "Race, gender, and partnership in the patient-physician relationship," *JAMA*, 282(6) (1999): 583–589.

Cross, T., Bazron, B. J., Dennis, K. W., & Isaacs, M. R., *Towards a Culturally Competent System of Care.* vol. 1: Monograph on effective services for minority children who are severely emotionally disturbed. (Washington, D.C.: CASSP Technical Assistance Center, Georgetown University Child Development Center (1989).

DuBard, C.A., & Massing, M.W., "Trends in emergency Medicaid expenditures for recent and undocumented immigrants," *JAMA* 297 (2007);1085–1092.

Flegal ,K.M., Carroll, M.D., Ogden C.L., & Johnson, C.L., "Prevalence and trends in obesity among U.S. adults, 1999–2000. *JAMA* 288 (2002):1723–1727.

Goldman, D.P., Smith, J.P., & Sood, N., "Immigrants and the cost of medical care," *Health Affairs*(Millwood) 25 (2006):1700–1711.

Grant, C., & Ladson-Billings, G. (eds.). *Dictionary of Multicultural Education.* (Phoenix: Oryx Press, 1997).

Hannan, E., Van Ryn, M., Burke, J., Stone, D., Kumar, D., Arani, D., Pierce, W., Rafi, S., Sanborn, T., Sharma, S., Slater, J., & DeBuono, B., "Access to coronary artery bypass surgery by race/ethnicity and gender among patients who are appropriate for surgery," *Medical Care* 37 (1999): 68–77.

Harris, L., Mungai, S., & Tierny, W., "Satisfaction with care in minority patients," in C. Hogue, M. Hargraves, & K. Collins (eds.), .*Minority Health in America: Findings and Policy Implications from the Commonwealth Fund Minority Health Survey*, (Baltimore: The John Hopkins University Press, 2000).

Herholz, H., Goff, D., Ramse, D., Chan, F., Ortiz, C., Labarthe, D., & Nichaman, M "Women and Mexican Americans receive fewer cardiovascular drugs following myocardial infarction than men and non-Hispanic whites: The Corpus Christi Heart Project, 1988–1990," *Journal of Clinical Epidemiology*, 49(3) (1996): 279–287.

Hogue, C., "Eating well, exercising and avoiding smoking: Health promotion among men and women in minority populations, in C. Hogue, M. Hargraves, & K. Collins (eds.), *Minority Health in America: Findings and Policy Implications from the Commonwealth Fund Minority Health Survey* (Baltimore: The John Hopkins University Press, 2000).

Hogue, C., & Hargraves, M., "The commonwealth fund minority health survey of 1994: An overview, in C. Hogue, M. Hargraves, & K. Collins, *Minority Health in America: Findings and Policy Implications from the Commonwealth Fund Minority Health Survey* (Baltimore: The John Hopkins University Press (2000).

Institute of Medicine, "Unequal treatment confronting racial and ethnic disparities in healthcare," *Institute of Medicine Report* (Washington, D.C.: National Academy Press, (2002).

Jones, J.H., *Bad Blood: The Tuskegee Syphilis Experiment*, expanded ed., (New York: Free Press, 1993).

Jones, J.H. *Bad blood: The Tuskegee syphilis experiment*, (New York: Macmillan, 1981).

Lancaster K.J., Watts, S.O., Dixon, L.B., "Dietary intake and risk of coronary heart disease differ among ethnic subgroups of black Americans," *J Nutr.* 136 (2006):446–451.

Late, M., & Krisberg, K., "Hurricane Katrina creates public health crisis on U.S. Gulf Coast: Health, medical workers responding," *Nation's Health* 35(8) (2005): 2005 American Public Health Association

Leonard, T,. "Exploring cultural, ethnic and racial diversity in baccalaureate nursing education programs," unpublished dissertation (Georgia State University: Atlanta, (2001).

McKinnon, J., "The black population in the United States: March 2000," *US Census 2000 Bureau, Current Population Reports,* Series P20–541. Available at http://www.census.gov/prod/2003pubs/p20-541.pdf.

Mohanty, S.A., Woolhandler, S., Himmelstein, D.U., Pati, S., Carrasquillo, O., Bor, & D.H., "Health care expenditures of immigrants in the United States: A nationally representative analysis," *Am J Public Health* 95 (2005): 1431–1438.

National Institutes of Health. *Women of color health data book*. Office of the Director, Publication No.02–4247, (Washington, D.C.: Author (2002).

New York City Department of Health and Mental Hygiene, *The Health of Immigrants in New York City,* (New York: Author, June 2006).

Pear, R., "Lacking papers, citizens are cut from Medicaid," *New York Times,* March 12, 2007, A1.

Satcher, D., *U.S. Public Health Service, Department of Health and Human Services Before the House Commerce Committee*, Report from the Subcommittee on Health and Environment (Washington, D.C.: U.S. Public Health Service, Department of Health and Human Services, May 11, 2000).

Satel, S., "Race for the cure: Does racism make you sick? *The New Republic*, 216(7) (1997): 12–13.

Smedley, B.D., Stith, A.Y., & Nelson, A.R., *Unequal treatment: Confronting racial and ethnic disparities in health care.* Institute of Medicine Report. (Washington, D.C.: National Academy Press, 2002).

Smith, D. B., *Health care divided: Race and healing a nation*. (Ann Arbor: The University of Michigan Press, 1999).

Smith, L., "Are we reaching the healthcare consumer?" *Journal of Cultural Diversity*, 5(2) (1997): 48–52.

Society for Women's Health Research, <www.womens-health.org>.

U.S. Department of Health and Human Services, *A Century of Women's Health: 1900–2000,* Office of Women's Health, (Washington, D.C.: Author, 2002).

U.S. Department of Commerce, Bureau of the Census, *Statistical Abstract of the United States* (Washington, D.C.: U.S. Government Printing Office, 2000).

U.S. Bureau of the Census, *Statistical Abstract of the United States* (Washington, D.C.: U.S. Government Printing Office, 2000).

U.S. Department of Health and Human Services, *Healthy People 2010: National Health Promotion and Disease Prevention Objectives* (Conference ed. in two vols.), Washington, D.C.: Author, 2000).

United States Kaiser Commission on Medicaid and the Uninsured, *Covering New Americans: A Review of Federal and State Policies Related to Immigrants' Eligibility and Access to Publicily Funded Health Insurance.* Shawn Fremstad and Laura Cox of the Center on Budget and Policy Priorities. November 2004.

Ward E., Jemal A., Cokkinides, V., Singh, G.K., Cardinez, C., Ghafoor, A., et al. "Cancer disparities by race/ethnicity and socioeconomic status," *CA Cancer J Clin.* 54 (2004):78–93.

Williams, D. R., "Race, socioeconomic status and health: The added effects of racism and discrimination," *Annals of the New York Academy of Sciences* 896 (1999): 173–188.

www.hud user.org/publications/ povsoc/annual.assess.html, Report on the homeless in the U.S.

Chapter 5

NUTRITION

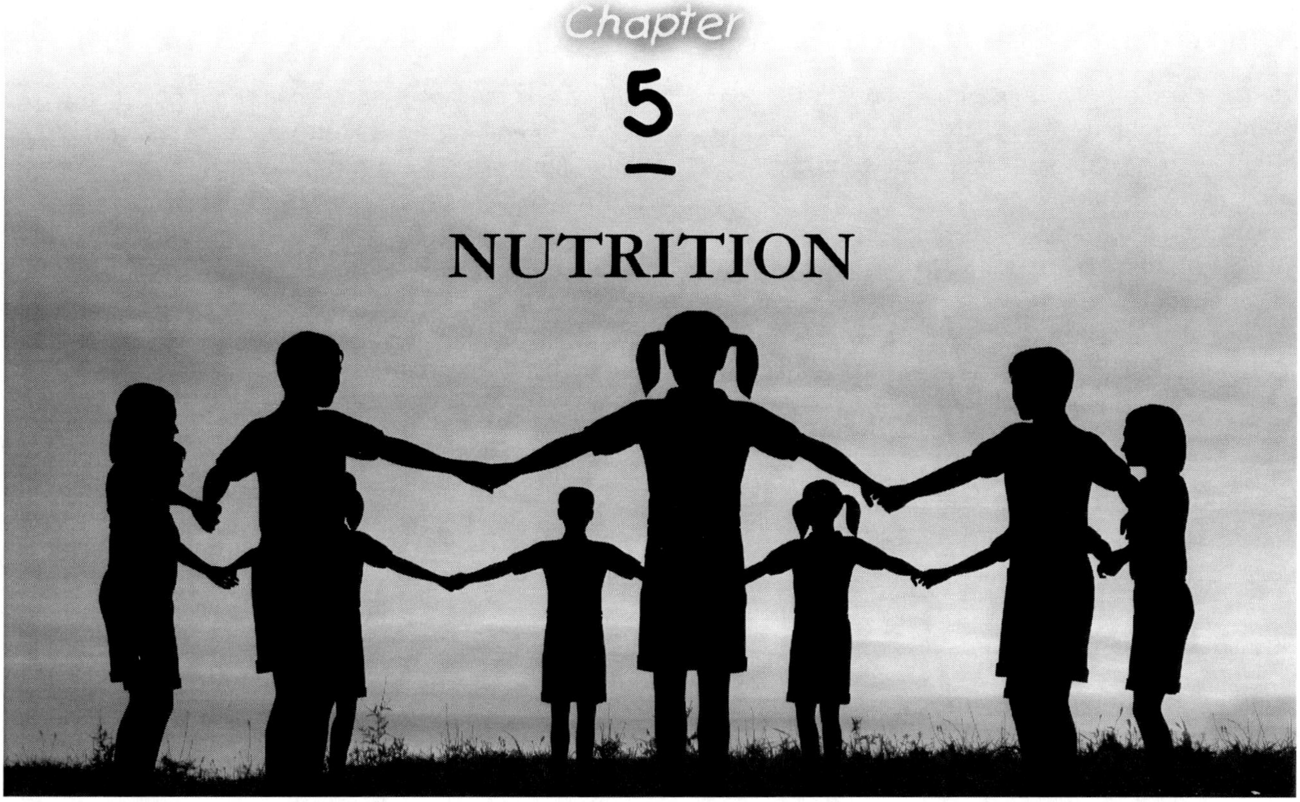

"Let food be your medicine."

—Hippocrates, the "father" of medicine

Food is among the most important things that people buy throughout their lives, and yet most people don't bother to take the time to find out exactly what is in the food that they buy and consume, where it comes from, or what chemical preservatives might have been added to it. All of the food that a person eats enters the body and becomes part of that person, thereby becoming a major determinant of the person's health status. Food affects whether a person is thin or fat, strong or weak, energetic or sluggish, and whether the person will die at a young age or live a long and healthy life. Americans today are bombarded with a vast array of choices and all too often make the mistake of buying food that is toxic. Much of the food produced and sold in the United States is contaminated by toxins, especially in the form of pesticides. In addition, harmful bacteria often enter the food supply from the ways in the food is grown, harvested, and processed.

The Bitter Truth About Fast Food

The fast food industry in the United States makes billions of dollars every year, despite growing concerns about the increasing rates of obesity, even among children, as well as increasing incidences of food poisoning. Studies have shown that Americans currently spend more money on fast food than they do on higher education, cars, personal computers, books, magazines, videos, and CDs. One survey found that 96% of young American children could identify Ronald McDonald, and that the golden arches that symbolize McDonald's was more widely recognized than the Christian cross.

Why does a fast food meal taste so good—unlike the meals that my mom makes?

Fast food tastes good partly because of added ingredients such as chemicals, "natural" and artificial flavors, and even food coloring. Studies indicate that such additives can have a significant effect on how a person perceives the taste of food. In addition, some of the chemicals added to fast food are actually addictive, which helps to explain why many adults who have regularly eaten fast food since they were children cannot simply quit eating it; they actually experience withdrawal symptoms when they go without it.

For these and other reasons, it is important that people carefully read the labels on the foods that they choose. The terms "natural flavor" and "artificial flavor" on food labels refer to human-made additives that enhance the taste of most processed foods. Commercials suggesting that people cannot stop after eating just a few potato chips are not far off the mark; it is very difficult for most people to stop because of the addictive ingredients and flavor enhancers that have been added to chips and other similar snacks. Coloring agents are added to many soft drinks, salad dressings, condiments, chicken dishes, cookies, bread, and other baked products. The Food and Drug Administration (FDA) does not require the manufacturers of food flavorings to disclose the ingredients in the flavorings, as long as all the chemicals that they contain are considered by the FDA to be "generally regarded as safe" (GRAS). This lack of a requirement to publically disclose ingredients allows enables the manufacturers to maintain the secrecy of their formulas.

Example of a widespread coloring agent

Do you eat strawberry yogurt, milkshakes, or frozen fruit bars? If so, you have probably been eating insects, too. Cochineal extract (also known as carmine or carminic acid) is a dye made from the dried crushed and bodies of the female *Dactylopius coccus*, or cochineal, a small insect that is harvested in Peru, the Canary Islands, Chile, and Mexico. Cochineals eat red cactus berries. The carmine color from the berries accumulates in the bodies of the females and in their unhatched larvae, producing the carmine dye. In addition to yogurt, frozen fruit bars, and milkshakes, some other sweets, fruit fillings, and juice drinks also get their pink color from carmine, therefore read the labels carefully.

Meat

Hamburgers

Hamburgers are one of the most popular foods worldwide. Countless cows are needed to produce the millions of hamburgers that are consumed daily throughout the world, and turning that much cattle into such a huge amount of beef meat requires large-scale industrial processes. A huge number of resources are needed to raise cattle, including land resources, water, soybeans, and grain to feed the cattle, which is often produced by chemical intensive-farming. It takes about 2,500 gallons of water and 16 pounds of grain and soybeans to produce just a single pound of hamburger. Multiplying these numbers by the estimated 67 to 69 pounds of beef that an average meat-eating American consumes per year adds up to an enormous amount of resources. In South America, huge areas of tropical rain forests have been cleared to make room for grazing land for cattle. The continuing destruction of rain forests is extinguishing countless and as yet undiscovered species of plants that could be medicinally beneficial to humans, not to mention the increased potential for global warming that the destruction of rain-forests is creating.

Other Meat Products

According to many scientists and researchers, meat products are becoming increasingly dangerous as a result of the way in which animals are raised and slaughtered. They often are confined to tiny cages crowded together, enabling illnesses and infections to be easily passed on from one animal to another. As a result, industrial farms frequently resort to the use of antibiotics to prevent the animals from becoming ill or diseased. It is not uncommon for industrial meat producers to slaughter numerous animals at one time and mix their meat together.

Although hogs produce three times the amount of fecal waste that humans do, hog farms are not required to treat the sewage of their animals. Instead, hog waste is typically stored in large ponds called lagoons.

According to Eric Schlosser, who investigated slaughterhouses for his book and movie *Fast Food Nation,* hog lagoons filled with waste can be as extensive as 20 acres and as deep as 15 feet. Dangerous chemicals, including hydrogen sulfide and ammonia, emanate from the lagoons. Some studies suggest that when humans breathe air polluted with hydrogen sulfide over a certain period of time, permanent damage to the nervous system and the brain can result. Moreover, the liquid waste from the lagoons is regularly sprayed onto fields, where it infests the soil with bacteria and toxins. Groundwater and nearby streams are commonly poisoned by the leakage and the overflowing of hog lagoons, and there are dead zones in the rivers downstream from these factory farms.

The huge slaughterhouses in which the animals are killed are dangerous and disturbing environments as well. The unskilled labor of meatpacking is both dirty and dangerous, and few slaughterhouses are unionized. Many of the workers in slaughterhouses are recent immigrants and illegal aliens. As for the animals, when cattle are driven through a chute into a slaughterhouse, a worker called a knocker shoots each steer in the head with a stun-gun that drives a retractable steel bolt into its brain. Once the animal has fallen lifelessly to the ground, another worker fastens a chain and hook attached to a pulley around one of the steer's rear legs, and the steer is then hauled upside down into the air. A worker called a sticker then slits the unconscious animal's throat—about once every ten seconds. The carcass then moves on down the disassembly line past other workers, with chain-saws, hooks, and knives, who carve it up into the parts to be sold for retail. Modern slaughterhouses can process thousands of heads of cattle in one day in this manner, resulting in the production of about 800,000 pounds of hamburger meat. It is entirely possible that the meat in a single fast-food hamburger could have come from dozens—or even hundreds—of steers.

The waste from the cattle carcasses in a slaughterhouse is rendered, or melted down, into a mixture of meat and bone meal. This mixture is used to make food for other animals to help them grow larger and more quickly. Animals that are raised for their meat or dairy products are also given growth hormones and steroids so as to maximize their growth and therefore their market value in the shortest possible period of time. Large amounts of antibiotics are also used to prevent diseases from spreading throughout a population of overcrowded animals, which has the negative consequence of creating drug-resistant bacteria in humans. Essentially, when humans eat the meat of animals that have been given hormones, steroids, and/or antibiotics, they are ingesting secondhand all of these substances themselves. This too can have harmful effects on the health of humans who eat the meat of these animals, including the potential to cause disease.

Two of the hormones that the meat industry uses, estradiol and zeranol, are likely to have harmful effects on humans, including cancer and hormonal changes. Concerns about these potential health impacts have caused many scientists to doubt the safety of hormone use in meat production.

Poultry litter is another type of animal feed made from biological waste. Poultry litter is a mixture of chicken excrement, spilled feed, dirt, feathers, and everything else that is scooped up from the floors of poultry sheds. Because poultry litter is much less expensive than plant crops are, the cattle industry in the United States feeds approximately one million tons of poultry litter to cattle every year.

Red Meat Increases the Risk of Cancer and Heart Attack

According to a study conducted by the National Institutes of Health in 2009 of more than 500,000 people, a diet that includes a high amount of red or processed meat can increase the risk of heart attacks in humans by 16% to 36% and cancers by 12% to 22%. Replacing red and processed with lean cuts of turkey and chicken can significantly decrease the risk of heart attacks and cancer.

rBGH/Hormones

Another problem with the meat industry, as well as the dairy industry, in the United States, is recombinant Bovine Growth Hormone (rBGH), which is a genetically engineered copy of a hormone that is naturally produced by cows and manufactured by Monsanto Company.

When rBGH is injected into dairy cows, it speeds up their production of milk, but at the same time, it makes them ill. These cows are at increased risk for developing udder infections, problems with reproduction, digestive disorders, hoof and leg ailments, and sores that don't heal properly. When these conditions develop, the cows are treated with antibiotics, a problem that was discussed earlier.

Even though rBGH has been banned in Europe and Canada and has been boycotted by about 95 percent of dairy farmers in the United States, the Food and Drug Administration (FDA), the Environmental Protection Agency, and the Department of Agriculture all license rBGH (as well as foods that are genetically engineered) without its having undergone safety testing. Pressure from the industry has allowed the sale of genetically engineered foods without a requirement that this be indicated on identifying labels.

Chicken

Many chickens in the United States are raised for their meat, in part because of the increasing demand for such fast-food products as chicken nuggets. As with cattle, chickens are given growth hormones. Often, these chickens grow so quickly that their legs cannot support the weight of their bodies. Most chickens, as well as turkeys and pigs that are raised on factory farms are confined to tiny pens or cages until they are taken to slaughter; they are never allowed the experiences of roaming freely, seeing daylight, or experiencing fresh air.

Even chicks are given hormones, as well as antibiotics, which are mixed in with their feed. This causes the chicks to grow very quickly, but it also causes their reproductive systems to develop prematurely. The result is a quick, unnatural burst of egg production, which wears out the chickens prematurely. In addition, the onslaught of hormones eventually overwhelms the chickens' livers, and the animals usually develop cancer of the liver within about 20 months. The chickens are sent to a slaughter house when their useful lives are over, just before liver cancer can be detected.

Chickens that have been given hormones and antibiotics usually begin laying eggs when they are about 5 months old. In contrast, chickens that are raised naturally and provided with healthy feed do not begin to lay eggs until they are at least 10 to 12 months old. They also usually live at least twice as long as chickens that are given hormones and antibiotics.

The most commonly used additive in chicken feed is oxarsone, which contains arsenic. Oxarsone promotes growth, kills parasites, and enhances the color of chicken meat. It is usually harmless, but under certain conditions, the oxarsone can be converted into more toxic forms of inorganic arsenic within the chickens' bodies or on farmland. Arsenic has been associated with a variety of cancers, such as bladder, lung, skin, kidney, and colon cancers. In addition, even low levels of exposure to arsenic can lead to partial paralysis and diabetes.

In one study, researchers randomly selected 407 processed chickens from 26 stores in Georgia, Maryland, Minnesota, and Oregon. The researchers found that more than half were tainted with antibiotic-resistant bacteria.

Chicken McNuggets

The name "Chicken McNugget" is a bit of an exaggeration. In fact, a chicken McNugget is made up of about 56% corn and thirty-eight other ingredients besides chicken. The most disturbing ingredient in Chicken McNuggets is tertiary butylhydroquinone (TBHQ), an antioxidant that is derived from petroleum. TBHQ is either sprayed directly on the nuggets or on the inside of the boxes that they are put into to "help preserve freshness." According to *A Consumer's Dictionary of Food Additives*, TBHQ is a form of butane (i.e., lighter fluid). Still, the FDA allows food processors to use it sparingly in food intended for human consumption. TBHQ can make up no more than 0.02% of the oil in a single nugget of chicken. However, if a person ingests just a single gram of TBHQ, it can cause nausea, vomiting, delirium, a feeling of suffocation, and even the collapse of the person. If a person ingests 5 grams of TBHQ, it can be fatal.

In addition to TBHQ, the fat content of chicken nuggets is a concern. Between 50% and 60% of the calories in most chicken nuggets comes from fat. The popularity of high-fat, highly processed fast foods, including chicken nuggets, is one of the reasons why the percentage of American children who are overweight has tripled in the past 20 years. Following is McDonald's own nutritional breakdown of a typical serving of Chicken McNuggets:

Ingredients:

White boneless chicken, water, food starch-modified, salt, chicken flavor (autolyzed yeast extract, salt, wheat starch, natural flavoring (botanical source), safflower oil, dextrose, citric acid, rosemary), sodium phosphates, seasoning (canola oil, mono- and diglycerides, natural extractives of rosemary). Battered and breaded with: water, enriched flour (bleached wheat flour, niacin, reduced iron, thiamin mononitrate, riboflavin, folic acid), yellow corn flour, food starch-modified, salt, leavening (baking soda, sodium acid pyrophosphate, sodium aluminum phosphate, monocalcium phosphate, calcium lactate), spices, wheat starch, whey, corn starch. Prepared in vegetable oil ((may contain one of the following: Canola oil, corn oil, soybean oil, hydrogenated soybean oil, partially hydrogenated soybean oil, *partially hydrogenated corn oil with TBHQ and citric acid added to preserve freshness), dimethylpolysiloxane added as an antifoaming agent). CONTAINS: WHEAT AND MILK

Nutrition Facts:

Serving size: 6 nuggets

Calories: 310

Fat calories: 180

Fat: 20 grams

Carbs: 18 grams

Protein: 15 grams

Percentage fat: 58%

(Source: McDonald's USA Ingredients http://www.mcdonalds.com/)

What you can do

Clearly, millions of animals caught within the process of factory farming suffer. If you don't want to be a part of this, you can switch to free-range or organic meat products. Organic chicken meat, especially meat from chickens raised on farms near where you live, is the most healthful choice. Organic chickens are better fed, less exposed to pesticides and harmful chemicals, and exposed to some sunlight, all of which makes them more healthful for human consumption. If you like chicken nuggets, stop eating the fast-food version and, instead, make them yourself and help improve your health. A recipe for healthful chicken nuggets is provided below.

Make Your Own Healthful Chicken Nuggets:

Ingredients:

1 cup dry bread crumbs

¼ cup parmesan cheese

2 tsp dried oregano

2 tsp dried basil

1 tsp paprika

½ tsp dried thyme

1½ lb. boneless, skinless chicken breasts, cup into 2-inch cubes

1 tbsp olive oil

*partially hydrogenated = trans fat

Instructions:

1. Preheat oven to 350 degrees.
2. In a large plastic bag, mix together all the ingredients except the chicken and oil.
3. After mixing together the ingredients, add the chicken cubes to the plastic bag and shake well.
4. On a nonstick cookie sheet, place the chicken cubes.
5. Either lightly spray olive oil from a bottle or sprinkle olive oil over the chicken.
6. Bake the chicken cubes for about 10 minutes, or until they are fully cooked.

Nutritional Information:

Calories: 239

Calories from Fat: 64

Total Fat: 7 g

Cholesterol: 71 mg

Sodium: 275 mg

Carbohydrate: 13 g

Dietary Fiber: 1 g

Sugar: 1 g

Protein: 29 g

McDonald's French Fries

In June of 2002, the McDonald's corporation was forced to pay $10 million to Hindu and vegetarian groups in the United States because it had misled the public about its french fries being vegetarian. Hindus do not eat beef for religious reasons. The groups of Hindus and vegetarians involved in the lawsuit against McDonald's had eaten french fries that had been pre-cooked in beef tallow, which McDonald's had described as "natural flavoring."

McDonald's described the production of its french fries on its Web site in January of 2003 in the following way: *"A small amount of beef flavoring is added during potato processing—at the plant. After the potatoes are washed and steam-peeled, they are cut, blanched, dried, par-fried, and frozen. It is during the par-frying process at the plant that the natural flavoring is used. These fries are then shipped to our U.S. restaurants. Our french fries are cooked in vegetable oil at our restaurants."*

In September of 2002, McDonald's pledged to start using a new oil that would contain half the level of harmful trans-fatty acids in its french fries as before. However, the company delayed those plans, citing product quality and customer satisfaction as priorities while testing of new oils continued. As a result of new and improved testing, in 2006, it was found that McDonald's french fries contained a third more trans fats than had previously been thought. This finding was based on the results of a new testing method that the company had begun to use the previous year. The conclusion is that the amount of potentially artery-clogging trans fats in a large serving of french fries is actually 8 grams, not the previously reported 6 grams, meaning that the total amount of fat contained in a large serving is actually 30 grams, not 25.

Concerns About Acrylamide

Acrylamide is a chemical that is produced during the frying, baking, or grilling of nearly all carbohydrate-rich foods especially fast-food french fries. Many scientists believe that acrylamide can cause nervous tremors in people who ingest the chemical in high amounts, and it has been associated with birth defects, male infertility, and cancer in lab animals. California's attorney general has joined a suit against McDonald's and other fast-food chains to require them to label their french fries accordingly. Following is McDonald's own nutritional breakdown of a typical serving of its french fries:

Ingredients:

Potatoes, vegetable oil (partially hydrogenated soybean oil, natural beef flavor (wheat and milk derivatives)*, citric acid (preservative), dextrose, sodium acid pyrophosphate (maintain color), dimethylpolysiloxane (antifoaming agent)), salt. Prepared in vegetable oil ((may contain one of the following: Canola oil, corn oil, soybean oil, hydrogenated soybean oil, **partially** hydrogenated soybean oil, partially hydrogenated corn oil with TBHQ and citric acid added to preserve freshness), dimethylpolysiloxane added as an antifoaming agent). (Natural beef flavor contains hydrolyzed wheat and hydrolyzed milk as starting ingredients.)

Nutrition Facts (Serving Size: 1 large order)

Total Fat: 30.0 g

Saturated Fat: 6.0 g; 46% of DV

Carbs: 70.0 g

Sodium: 330 mg

Calories from Fat: 270

Calories: 570

Protein: 6.0 g

1 lb russet potatoes

1 quart chilled water

1 tray of ice cubes

1/2 tsp salt

Spray Canola oil

(Source: McDonald's USA Ingredients http://www.mcdonalds.com/)

Make Your Own Healthful French Fries

Ingredients:

potatoes

salt

canola oil

1. Peel and slice potatoes, then place them in a mixing bowl with cold water and ice cubes. Soak for 30 minutes. Preheat oven to 400°F.
2. After soaking the potatoes, drain them and then pat them dry with a paper towel.
3. Place the potatoes and salt in a plastic zipper bag. Spray the potatoes for about 3 seconds with canola oil, and then seal the plastic zipper bag. Shake to coat the potatoes well with the oil and salt.
4. Carefully place the potatoes on a non-stick cookie sheet so that they don't touch one another. Spray lightly with canola oil.
5. Place the cookie sheet in the oven and allow the potatoes to bake for about 7 minutes. Turn the potatoes at least twice, cooking for about 7 minutes after each turn. The total cooking time is 20–25 minutes.

*CONTAINS: WHEAT AND MILK

Nutrition Facts

Calories: 86

Total Fat: 0 g

Saturated Fat: 0 g

Trans Fat: 0 g

Cholesterol: 0 mg

Sodium: 297 mg

Total Carbohydrates: 20 g

Dietary Fiber: 2 g

Sugars: 1 g

Protein: 2 g

Contaminated Fish

Fish and seafood farming is the fastest growing sector of food production in the world—and one of the fastest growing threats to marine environments and their native species. There are health and food-safety concerns about human consumption of farm-bred fish. Fish that have been farmed often are given large doses of antibiotics to protect them from diseases. They also are exposed to a number of pesticides that kill parasites and body fungi, all of which accumulate in the tissues of the fish. When people eat this fish, they also ingest traces of the pesticides, which can remain in the internal organs.

The most common farm-raised fish include catfish, salmon, trout, and shrimp. When you buy fish, make sure to read the labels or ask an employee whether the fish is wild or farm raised. Choose wild fish to help protect your health.

Mercury pollution is another concern about human consumption of fish. Mercury from coal-fired power plants is absorbed into the air, deposited in bodies of water through natural weather processes, and enters the skin of fish. The fish that are most commonly contaminated with mercury include tuna, sea bass, farm-raised salmon, swordfish, shark, tilefish, and king mackerel. Other fish and shellfish that are tainted with mercury, but in lower amounts, include sea bass, marlin, halibut, pike, walleye, white croaker, largemouth bass, and oysters from the Gulf of Mexico. A pregnant woman who consumes mercury via contaminated fish can pass it on to her fetus through the placenta, with the potential of damaging the brain of the fetus. This can lead later on to learning disabilities, the delay of the mental development of the child, and other neurological problems.

It was recently reported that some people in New York City have been fishing in the Hudson River due to economic hardships, but unfortunately all of the fish that these people caught was found to be contaminated with deadly chemicals.

Globalization and Food Safety

Globalization is the increasing flow of money, goods, services, and people across national borders. Globalization has had both positive and negative impacts on communities throughout the world. Many people have been lifted from poverty as more jobs have become available; however, in many cases, globalization has contributed to the greater marginalization of poor people, who do not have access to essential goods such as life-saving medicine and safe food.

Ensuring the safety of the world's food supply has become increasingly difficult as a result of globalization. In addition, the incidences of food-borne illnesses are likely to increase because of the ways in which food is grown and processed. ***Every two hours, one person in the United States dies from contaminated food.***

In the beginning of the 1900s, the majority of people in the United States were farmers. Today, farmers make up less than 2% of the population in the United States. Much of the food produced in this country is grown by large agricultural corporations whose main interests are to maximize their profits. The result is that petrochemicals, drugs, artificial fertilizers, and toxic pesticides are used on crops, which can have harmful effects on the health of people who consume them.

As a result of globalization, it is now cheaper for food processing companies to buy ingredients from countries that sell these ingredients at lower costs than those found in the United States. In recent years, there has been an international outbreak of *E. coli* poisoning from fresh spinach, as well as a major recall of pet food as a result of numerous deaths of cats and dogs. In the case of the contaminated spinach, which occurred in the fall of 2006, more than 200 people in the United States and Canada became ill after eating fresh-cut spinach from a single producer.

In recent years, food products ranging from eggs to pork that were tainted with dioxin (an industrial chemical) were exported from Belgium to other European countries, as well as to North America, Australia, and New Zealand. In 2008, many Chinese babies had to be attached to life-saving dialysis machines after consuming contaminated formula that contained melamine, a chemical used in the manufacture of different kinds of industrial products. Melamine is used in combination with formaldehyde in the manufacture of plastics and cleaning products. It is also combined with other chemicals in the production of fire retardants, pesticides, fertilizers, and concrete. In 2007, an estimated 4,100 cats and dogs in the United States died of kidney failure caused by the formation of renal crystals or kidney stones. The cause of renal toxicity was traced back to melamine that was detected in pet food.

The Centers for Disease Control and Prevention has reported that an estimated 76 million cases of food-borne illnesses occur every year in the United States. Of these cases, about 325,000 require hospitalization, and about 5,000 result in death. More Americans die every year from what they eat than were killed in the terrorist attacks of September 11, 2001.

The two most common illness caused by contaminated food are salmonella and *E coli.* These bacteria are deadly because they are found in the fecal matter of factory-farm animals. The ways in which meat is processed after the animals are slaughtered spreads the fecal matter to the meat and then into people's bodies.

The three federal agencies that regulate food safety in the United States are

1. The Food and Drug Administration (FDA),
2. The Department of Agriculture (USDA), and
3. The Environmental Protection Agency (EPA).

Some of the most common food-borne illnesses that affect humans include the following:

Botulism is a rare illness caused by the bacterium *Clostridium botulinum,* which produces botulin, a toxin that attacks the nerves and can lead to paralysis and death. **Symptoms:** double vision, difficulty swallowing, slurred speech, and muscle weakness, all of which usually appear within 18 to 36 hours of infection but can begin as soon as six hours or as late as ten days after infection.

Sources: improperly canned foods, garlic and herbs preserved in oil, vacuum-packed and tightly wrapped foods, lunch meats, ham, sausage, smoked and salted fish, and honey.

Prevention: Do not eat food from bulging or dented cans; use hygienic methods of home canning, including boiling home-canned foods for at least 10 minutes.

Listeriosis is an illness caused by *Listeria monocytogenes,* a bacterium found in water and soil, and often carried by animals. Pregnant women account for about one-third of all cases of listeriosis, which can lead to miscarriage or stillbirth, premature delivery, or the infection or death of the newborn.

Symptoms: a flu like fever and muscle aches, which usually begin within 48 to 72 hours of infection but can appear as long as 7 to 30 days later. If the infection spreads to the nervous system, the person's symptoms might also include a stiff neck, headache, nausea, and vomiting.

Sources: soft cheeses; unpasteurized dairy products, raw or undercooked meat, hot dogs, poultry, lunch meats, dried sausage, meat spreads, and smoked seafood.

Salmonella is a diarrheal infection caused by Salmonella bacteria, which are usually transmitted to humans foods contaminated with animal feces.

Symptoms: diarrhea, fever, and abdominal cramps, usually 12 to 72 hours after infection.

Sources: contaminated foods from an animal origin; these foods include beef, poultry, milk, and eggs. However, any type of food, including fruits and vegetables, can become contaminated. Raw eggs are often a source of infection, but people can be unaware that they are eating them when they are used in such home-made foods as hollandaise sauce, caesar and other salad dressings, tiramisu, ice cream, mayonnaise, cookie dough, and frosting.

Toxoplasmosis is an infection caused by the *Toxoplasma gondii* parasite which usually affects people with weak immune systems. Although more than 60 million people in the United States might be carrying this parasite, most have immune system that are healthy enough to prevent it from causing them to become ill.

Symptoms: Swollen lymph glands and muscle aches within a week to a month after infection, which can last for a month or more but also can remain dormant. As the infection travels though the bloodstream of a person with a weak immune system, toxoplasmosis can cause damage to the brain, eyes, and other organs. A small percentage of infected newborns have serious eye or brain damage.

Sources: Raw or undercooked meats (especially pork, lamb, and game), untreated water (in rivers and ponds), and parasite-infected cats.

Prevention: If you have a weakened immune system or are pregnant, wear clean latex gloves while handling raw meats, when gardening where cats may have defecated, and when handling litter boxes.

E coli Is a bacterial pathogen found in cattle and similar animals. People usually become infected with *E.coli* after consuming food or water that has been contaminated with microscopic amounts of cow feces.

Symptoms: Severe, bloody diarrhea and abdominal cramps, without much fever. Sometimes, a complication called hemolytic uremic syndrome (HUS) can arise weeks after the initial symptoms. These cases usually occur in very young children, the elderly, or those with weakened immune systems. HUS includes temporary anemia, extensive bleeding, and kidney failure.

Sources: Raw or undercooked ground beef, unpasteurized milk, some fresh produce such as alfalfa and radish sprouts, and unpasteurized apple juice and cider.

Mad Cow Disease In humans, this disease is called Creutzfeld-Jacob disease (CJD) and is very similar to Alzheimer's disease. CJD creates spongelike holes in an infected person's brain and is always fatal—there is no treatment or cure.

Symptoms: CJD earned the nickname "mad cow disease" because of the symptoms that affected cattle exhibitied, such as staggering, tremors, muscle spasms, bewilderment, and hypersensitivity to some stimuli. Because there is no blood test available for people who are alive, CJD has been diagnosed definitively only through brain biopsies.

Sources: Contaminated nerve tissue in cow-meat products such as hot dogs, salami, and pepperoni.

Prevention: If you eat beef, choose organic beef and beef products that are not likely to contain tissue from a cow's nervous system (such as the brain, spinal cord, and nerve endings), which is the most infectious part of a cow with the disease. Unfortunately, the risk of infection cannot be reduced by cooking beef more thoroughly, because, unlike bacteria and viruses, heat does not destroy the prions that cause mad cow disease.

In European countries, one of every four cows is tested for mad cow disease. In Japan 100% of cattle intended for human consumption is tested. In those countries, a number of cases of mad cow disease have been detected in animals that appeared to be perfectly healthy. In the United States, only about one of every 18,000 cows that have been slaughtered are tested. In addition, the type of testing methods that are used in the this country have been shown to miss prions that can be detected by the more-advanced testing methods used in Europe. Testing every cow in the United States that is intended for human consumption appears to be the only way to ensure the safety of the supply of beef. It has been estimated that the testing of every cow destined for slaughter would add only a few cents per pound to the cost of hamburger meat.

How to avoid food-borne illnesses:

The federal food safety agencies are failing to protect Americans from food-borne illnesses. Our government must be held accountable for ensuring that mandatory food-safety programs are implemented and that there are more frequent inspections of processing plants. For years, many people have been calling for the reorganization of the U.S. Department of Agriculture, the Food and Drug Administration, and other agencies and for the creation of a single, centralized food-inspection authority. The food-safety programs in this country are under-funded and under-staffed.

Presently, the best means of protection against food-borne infections is to take preventative measures, such as cooking meat to appropriate temperatures, avoiding cross-contamination between meat and other foods, preparing food using sanitary practices, and consuming only pasteurized milk, cheeses, and juices.

Preventative steps to decrease the risk of food-borne illnesses:

- Cook ground beef, pork, veal, and lamb to a uniform internal temperature of at least 160 °F and ground poultry to 165 °F. Cook beef, veal, and lamb meat cuts such as roasts to an internal temperature of at least 145 °F; pork meat cuts to 160 °F; and nonground poultry to 170 °F. Reheat these foods to 160 °F or until they are steaming hot. Keep hot foods at or above 140 °F and cold foods at or below 40 °F.
- Avoid drinking unpasteruized milk, apple juice, or cider.
- Wash hands thoroughly with soap and hot water after handling raw meat products to prevent cross-contamination of other foods.
- Wash hands often and thoroughly to help prevent person-to-person transmission.
- Drink water from public or clean well sources, never from untreated streams, ponds, or lakes.
- Wash fruits and vegetables thoroughly (even if the package indicated that is has been "triple washed") using clean, drinkable water, a vegetable and fruit cleaning product, or vinegar.
- Carefully follow instructions on food packages, including "Keep refrigerated," "Sell by . . . ," and "Use by . . ." dates.

Irradiation

Irradiation is the exposure of food to ionizing radiation for the purposes of disinfecting, sanitizing, sterilizing, and preserving it, or to eliminate the infestation of insects from food. Irradiation was approved in 2002 in the United States as a treatment for all pests in a small percentage of imported fruits and vegetables. In 2006, irradiation was approved for a wider range of food products, including an expanded number of fruits and vegetables, herbs and spices, wheat flour, white potatoes, pork, and poultry.

There is no government requirement that irradiated foods be labeled as such.

Irradiated food is bombarded with levels of radiation that are 5,000 to 1 million times greater than the level of radiation of a typical chest X-ray.

Many scientists are raising concerns about the possible effects of irradiated foods, which they suspect might destroy vital nutrients and vitamins, as well as alter the chemical structure of the foods. The health risks and long-term effects on human health of irradiated foods is as yet unknown.

The nonprofit public-interest group Public Citizen objects to the irradiation of foods. The group has stated that lab animals that ate irradiated foods developed serious health problems, including the following:

- premature death,
- fatal internal bleeding,
- a rare form of cancer,
- a high rate of stillbirths and other reproductive problems,
- mutations and other genetic damage,

- organ malfunctioning,
- stunted growth,
- vitamin deficiencies.

Genetically Engineered Foods

Genetic engineering is the process of modifying the genetic makeup of a live organism. In genetic engineering, scientists take genetic material from one organism and insert it into the permanent genetic code of another organism. Using this process, biotechnologists actually create new forms of organisms. Some examples of genetic engineering include tomatoes that have been altered to slow the softening process, strawberries that have been changed so that they are preserved better after freezing, potatoes that produce toxins to repel or kill pests, and soybeans that can tolerate chemical herbicides. Currently, approximately 40% of the corn and 80% of the soybeans grown in the United States are genetically engineered. Some health experts warn that foods produced by genetic engineering are hazardous to human health, and some environmental scientists are concerned that genetic engineering might upset the normal balance of ecosystems and the natural order of living things.

The affects of these unnaturally altered food products on human health and on the environment are largely unknown. The most common effect observed so far has been allergic reactions to the proteins added to genetically engineered foods in people who are not normally allergic to those particular foods.

Food Miles, Resources, and the Environment

As a result of globalization and industrialization, the world's food supplies today are grown and processed in fewer locations than ever, which means that the food must travel farther to reach consumers' homes. Although highly centralized food production is considered to be efficient and is certainly profitable for large agricultural businesses, many people believe that it is harmful to the environment, to consumers, and to rural communities.

Food miles are the distance that a food product travels from its source to the consumer's home. An estimated 80% of the energy used in the U.S. food system is consumed by the processing, packaging, transporting, storing, and preparing of food. About 40% of the fruit consumed in the United States is produced overseas; a typical fruit or vegetable that is purchased at a grocery store has traveled about 1,500 food miles.

What you can do

Buying food that is grown or produced locally significantly reduces food miles and therefore transportation costs, which conserves energy. Locally grown products are fresher, taste better, and are packed with more nutrition, which benefits consumers. Because these foods do not have to travel far, farmers can choose to grow varieties of foods based on flavor rather than on their ability to withstand long journeys to different markets. Knowing who is growing your food can be a powerful thing, and purchasing products from local farmers and food producers keeps more money in your community.

As a consumer, remember to also buy rBGH-free milk, cheese, yogurt, butter, ice-cream, infant formula, and meat. Try to buy organic foods as well as local foods.

Organic food is food that is produced by farmers who are committed to the use of renewable resources and the conservation of soil and water to preserve the quality of the environment for future generations. Organic meat, poultry, eggs, and dairy products come from animals that are raised without being given antibiotics or growth hormones. Organic produce is grown without the use of most conventional pesticides, without fertilizers made with synthetic ingredients or sewage sludge, without genetic engineering; and without irradiation. Before a food product can be labeled "organic," a person who is approved by the government inspects the farm where the food is grown to make sure that the farmer is following all the rules required to meet the USDA's organic standards.

"Natural" food is not the same as "organic" food. "Natural" can refer to one or more ingredients that are derived from a plant or animal and added for flavor, not nutrition. For example, mint ice-cream's "natural" flavor might refer to the mint that is added to the ice cream.

Guide to Organic Food Terms

When you buy organic foods, look for the "USDA Organic" label. Only foods in the categories "100% organic" and "organic" are permitted to display the USDA Organic Seal. In addition to the other requirements mentioned earlier, organic farmers must practice certain soil and water conservation methods and adhere to rules regarding the humane treatment of animals. The following terms related to organic foods are approved by the USDA:

- **"100% organic:"** a product is composed of a single ingredient, such as a fruit, vegetable, meat, milk, and cheese (excluding water and salt)
- **"Organic:"** a product contains multiple ingredients that are 95% to 100% organic
- **"Made with organic ingredients:"** 70% of the product's ingredients are organic
- **"Contains organic ingredients:"** a product is made up of less than 70% organic ingredients

Fair Trade Certified is a certification that ensures that farms in developing countries provide humane working conditions and reasonable wages for workers. Under this certification, farms must also use sustainable farming methods that protect the environment. This label most often is found on coffee, tea, chocolate, rice, sugar, grapes, and other fruit.

Certified Humane is a certification that ensures that animals have safe, healthful homes on farms and a diet that does not contain antibiotics or hormones. In addition, farmers comply with the standards for this certification to help prevent damage to land, air, and water. This label most often is found on eggs, beef, chicken, lamb, pork, and turkey.

Rainforest Alliance Certified is a certification that ensures that local cultures are preserved, that farmers treat workers fairly, and that the use of pesticides is minimal, thereby protecting water, soil, and tropical wildlife. This label most often is found on coffee, orange juice, chocolate, and bananas.

Free-range is a label for poultry that means the bird had access to the outdoors. Unfortunately, the time that a bird spends outside is not regulated, so that time could in fact be minimal.

Globesity

An average adult needs to consume a minimum of about 2,000 kilocalories a day. In simple terms, a person who takes in more calories than his or her body uses will gain weight.

Globesity is a blend of the terms *global* and *obesity.* It refers to the current global public-health crisis that is caused by excessive weight gain. **Obesity** is the condition of a proportionately high amount of excess body fat and is associated with a variety of debilitating and life-threatening disorders. Obesity is a complex condition, one with serious social and psychological dimensions, that today affects virtually all age and socioeconomic groups. Throughout the world, there are more than 1 billion overweight adults, with at least 300 million of them being obese. Rates of obesity rates have tripled since 1980 in some parts of North America, the United Kingdom, Eastern Europe, the Middle East, the Pacific Islands, Australia, and China. In South Africa, obesity rates are about equal to those of the United States, with one out of every three men and more than one out of every two adult women being overweight or obese. The epidemic of obesity is not restricted to the most developed countries, however; the rise in rates of obesity is faster in some developing countries than it is in developed countries.

Almost two-thirds of Americans are currently overweight, and approximately 300,000 Americans die every year of complications related to obesity. The problem of obesity is particularly worrisome because it now affects children even more so than adults, for example, by leading to the early onset of type 2 diabetes, which at one time was virtually never seen in children.

Major Factors for Globesity

1. An increase in consumption of high-energy, high-calorie foods
2. An increase in consumption of foods with few nutrients

3. An increase in consumption of high levels of fats and sugars
4. A decrease in levels of physical activity

The "toxic" environment of the modern world in which we live contributes to globesity. Some of the factors that contribute to globesity include the following:

- **Foods that lack nutrition are available everywhere and nearly anytime:** A large variety of high-fat, high-sugar foods is widely available. These foods taste good and cost less than more healthful foods do. There are strips of fast-food restaurants along America's highways and roads and rows of candy at the checkout counters of virtually all convenience and grocery stores.
- **Huge serving sizes :** There are many restaurants that serve all-you-can eat buffets, and many fast-food chains offer "value meals" that contain more food for less money.
- **Advertisements:** There is a barrage of advertising on television and in newspapers and magazines for prepackaged foods and fast-foods. Colorfully packaged single servings add to the appeal of processed foods.
- **Physical activity has declined in schools and recess time is being cut:** Most Americans get less exercise than ever before, while driving or riding in a car or other transportation more often than walking or riding bikes to even short destinations. Some studies show a direct link between watching more than 2 hours of TV and being overweight.

Americans spend $110 billion a year on fatty and sugary fast foods. Nearly every country in the world now has McDonald's and Pizza Hut restaurants, and Coca-Cola and Pepsi products have been distributed worldwide for many years.

The findings of a new study by the Centers for Disease Control and Prevention (CDC) and the Agency for Healthcare Research and Quality indicate that obesity is taking an incredible toll on the health-care system of the United States. The report found that the annual cost of obesity in the United States is an estimated $147 billion. The researchers involved based their analysis on data from 1998 and 2006 medical and health spending surveys. They defined *obesity* as a person having a body mass index above 30.

The body mass index (BMI) is a measure of body fat based on height and weight, and it applies both to adult men and women.

$$\text{BMI} = (\text{Weight in pounds} \div [\text{Height in inches}] \times [\text{Height in inches}]) \times 703$$

BMI Categories:

- **Underweight:** <18.5
- **Normal Weight:** 18.5–24.9
- **Overweight:** 25–29.9
- **Obese:** 30 or greater

Researchers in the study cited above found that the bulk of health-care spending related to obesity did not go towards treatments such as bariatric surgery, but instead went to treating diseases associated with obesity. They also noted that a significant amount of excess weight is the best predictor of a person's developing diabetes, the treatment of which accounts for approximately $191 billion annually.

Being overweight is a known risk factor for the following:

- diabetes,
- coronary heart disease,
- hypertension,
- stroke,
- high blood cholesterol,

- gallbladder disease,
- the degeneration of cartilage and bone in the joints,
- sleep apnea and other breathing problems, and
- cancers, including breast, colorectal, endometrial, and kidney cancer.

Obesity is also associated with the following:

- complications with pregnancy
- menstrual irregularities,
- excess body and facial hair,
- incontinence,
- psychological disorders such as depression,
- increased surgical risks, and
- increased mortality.

Solutions to reducing and preventing obesity:

Obesity is a disease largely caused by social and environmental factors, and it urgently needs to be addressed throughout the world. We need to develop strategies that will make it easier for people to make healthful choices. Effective weight management for people who are obese or are at risk of developing obesity requires a range of long-term strategies.

Nutritional experts have recommended the following community-based solutions for decreasing the epidemic of obesity:

- Develop supportive environments through public policies that make a wide variety of low-fat, high-fiber foods more available and accessible, and that provide opportunities for different types of physical activity.
- Promote healthful behaviors to motivate, encourage, and enable people to lose weight by
  - eating more fruits, vegetables, and whole grains;
  - exercising moderately every day for at least 30 minutes;
  - reducing the intake of fatty, sugary foods; and
  - eating unsaturated oil-based fats instead of trans fats and saturated animal-based fats.
- Make physical activities more accessible by building walking path and biking lanes, as well as more playgrounds that are safe.
- Sponsor and fund after-school recreational programs.
- Regulate advertising on television that is aimed at children and mandate equal time for pro-nutrition messages.
- Remove and ban fast foods and soft drinks from schools.
- Redesign school lunch programs to include more healthful food choices.
- Subsidize healthful foods to lower the prices of fruits and vegetables.

Undernutrition

You probably know what it's like to feel hungry even when you miss one meal.

Some children and adults are hungry almost all the time because they simply do not have enough food to eat, nor do they have safe drinking water. More than 3 billion people in the world are condemned to premature death from hunger and thirst. An estimated 1.5 billion people worldwide live on less than one dollar a day, and every 3.6 seconds, someone in the world dies of hunger. Hunger not only kills people, but it also deprives them of their ability to work and learn.

An estimated 35 million low-income Americans—about a third of which are children—cannot consistently afford to buy enough food. About 16% of people in the United Sates are regularly food insecure, which means that they don't have enough money to be sure that will be able to afford sufficient food throughout the year.

Causes of Undernutrition

- poverty,
- low educational level,
- scarceness of food because of drought or war,
- the existence of too many children in one family,
- contaminated food or water,
- diarrheal diseases, and
- dehydration.

Hunger versus Malnutrition

Hunger is a deficiency in caloric intake. Anyone whose daily diet provides them with fewer than the defined minimum of 2,000 kilocalories is considered to be suffering from hunger, or undernourishment. There are many organizations that help those suffering from hunger by providing food aid that supplements their daily caloric intake.

The World Health Organization estimates that there are 178 million malnourished children worldwide, and that, at any given time, 20 million people are suffering from the most severe form of malnutrition. Malnutrition is a factor in the deaths of between 3.5 and 5 million children who are under 5 years of age each year.

Malnutrition is the condition of having too little food or a severe lack of essential nutrients. Most food aid provided by nonprofit organizations is not an adequate response to malnutrition because it either contains insufficient amounts of essential nutrients or provides them in a way that cooking destroys them or they cannot be properly absorbed by the bodies of those who are malnourished.

When there are severe deficiencies in children's diets, their growth is stunted. This condition is called chronic malnutrition. When children experience weight loss, or are wasting away, they are suffering from acute malnutrition, which is classified into two main forms: severe wasting (marasmus) and nutritional edema (kwashiorkor). Marasmus is the condition of having an inadequate intake of calories and protein, whereas kwashiorkor is the condition of a having a fair-to-normal caloric intake but inadequate protein.

Signs and symptoms of protein-energy malnutrition include the following:

- little or no weight gain,
- the slowing of growth in height,
- behavioral changes such as apathy, irritability, decreased social responsiveness, anxiety, and attention deficits, and
- micronutrient deficiencies.

The most common and severe micronutrient deficiencies in children and childbearing women worldwide are deficiencies of iron, iodine, zinc, and vitamin A. Some fortification programs in the United States have helped diminish deficiencies of iodine and vitamin A in malnourished people; however, these deficiencies are still a significant cause of illnesses in developing countries. Micronutrient, protein, and calorie deficiencies need to be addressed for these people to achieve optimal growth and development.

The most common nutritional deficiencies and their symptoms include the following:

- **Iron:** fatigue, anemia, diminished cognitive functions, headaches, and changes in the nails
- **Iodine:** goiter, developmental delays, and mental retardation
- **Vitamin D:** slow growth, rickets, and hypocalcemia
- **Vitamin A:** night blindness, slow growth, and changes in the hair
- **Folate:** anemia, and neural tube defects in the fetuses of women who do not take folate supplements
- **Zinc:** anemia, dwarfism, lowered immune responses, problems with the healing of wounds

The Farm Bill is a U.S. law that is renewed about every five years and governs federal farm support, food stamps, agricultural trade, marketing, and rural development. Under the Farm Bill, the government makes large payments to farmers who produce a small number of crops. Most of the payments are for wheat, corn, cotton, rice, soybeans, sorghum, sugar, and dairy products. There is also support, but to a lesser extent, for peanuts, honey, chickpeas, dried beans, and wool. Unfortunately, farmers who grow fresh fruits and vegetables do not receive federal subsidies. This is why the real prices of fruits and vegetables increase, but the prices of soft drinks (made from high-fructose corn syrup) do not. One reason why some of the least healthful foods in grocery stores are the cheapest is that these foods are the ones for which the Farm Bill provides subsidies to farmers.

High-Fructose Corn Syrup

High-fructose corn syrup (HFCS) is made by changing the sugar glucose in cornstarch into another sugar, fructose. The end product is a combination of fructose and glucose. HFCS is used to extend the shelf-life of processed foods, and it is cheaper than sugar. HFCS is an ingredient that is widely used in many sodas, fruit-flavored drinks, and other processed foods.

According to the April 2004 issue of the *American Journal of Clinical Nutrition*, between 1970 and 1990, the consumption of HFCS in the United States increased by more than 1,000 percent. HFCS now accounts for more than 40% of calorie-containing sweeteners that are added to foods and beverages and is the only calorie-containing sweetener used in soft drinks in the United States.

Critics of HFCS say that it contributes to weight gain, tricks the body into wanting to eat more, and causes triglycerides to increase, which is an indicator of risk for cardiovascular disease. Many top health experts think that it is a dangerous chemical concoction.

> ***"If we can conquer space, we can conquer childhood hunger."***
>
> ***—Buzz Aldrin***

How to End Hunger

In the late 1960s and early 1970s, the U.S. government enacted a bipartisan plan to create and expand nutrition programs for children and the elderly. The end result was that hunger was nearly wiped out in the United States. However, over the past several years, the federal government's support for these programs has decreased, and the number of Americans who suffer from hunger has skyrocketed.

Some of the programs that were targeted budget cuts included the following:

- **Food stamps,** which help more than 25 million low-income people obtain the food necessary for their families to survive;
- **School breakfast and school lunch programs,** which provide free and low-cost meals to more than 22 million school children; and

- **The Special Supplemental Nutrition Program for Women, Infants, and Children, (WIC)**, which provides nutritious food, nutrition counseling, and health care referrals to about 8 million low-income women, infants, and children.

Using the tools of education, research, outreach, and advocacy, we must make a commitment to end hunger in this country. As a basic human right, all people should have the ability to buy safe and healthful food.

What you can do to help end hunger

- Call, write, or e-mail your elected representatives to encourage them to reduce hunger by improving and expanding national nutrition programs.
- Make a pledge to the International Alliance to End Hunger, an organization that is recording pledges to help end hunger from individuals, organizations, businesses, and nations. The organization's Web site is www.iaahp.net.
- Donate money to a local, national, or international nonprofit hunger organization; donate food to a local food bank; or volunteer to help at a local soup kitchen.
- Make www.thehungersite.com your home page and click on it every day; sponsors pay for food for the hungry with every hit.
- Visit the One Campaign's Web site at www.onecampaign.org and sign the One Campaign Declaration urging our government leaders to honor the Millennium Development Goals, and wear the white band to show others your support.
- Skip a meal for hunger and donate the cost of the meal to hunger organizations. Visit the Web site www.oxfamamerica.org.

Community interventions to help end hunger

- Make sure that states, localities, and schools offer all available federal food-assistance programs and work actively to enroll eligible people in these programs.
- Extend eligibility for food stamps to more people who have low incomes and are struggling.
- Increase access to children's nutrition programs so that more eligible children can benefit.
- Strengthen federal commodity food programs.
- Provide the WIC program with sufficient funds so that all eligible women, children, and infants can participate.
- Invest more in public education to increase outreach and awareness of the importance of preventing hunger and improving nutrition for health, learning, and productivity.
- Work to increase public awareness of the problem of hunger in the community and advocate for policies to end hunger.

References

Bock, S.A., "Prospective appraisal of complaints of adverse reactions to foods in children during the first 3 years of life," *Pediatrics* 79(19870: 683–688.

Centers for Disease Control and Prevention, "Preliminary FoodNet Data on the Incidence of Foodborne Illnesses—Selected Sites, United States, 1999," *MMWR* 49(2000): 210–205.

Centers for Disease Control and Prevention, "Summary of Notifiable Diseases, United States, 1999," *MMWR* 48 (2001): 1–104.

Council of Economic Advisers, "Economic Report of the President" (Washington, DC: Government Printing Office, 2006), Chapter 8, p. 179.

Chemical & Engineering News, vol. 85, No. 15, April 9, 2007: 34–35

Drabenstott, Mark, "Do Farm Payments Promote Rural Economic Development?" *The Main Street Economist,* March 2005.

Feder, B.J., "Biotech firm to advocate labels on genetically altered products," New York Times, February 24, 1997.

Food and Drug Administration, "Guidance for Industry: Questions and Answers, BSE Feed Regulation 21, *Code of Federal Regulations* 589, 2000.

Gould, F., Anderson, A., Jones, A., Sumerford, D., Heckel, D.G., Lopez, J., Micinski, S., Leonard, R., & M. Laster, "Initial frequency of alleles for resistance to *Bacillus Rhuringiensis* toxins in field populations of *Heliothis virescens,"* Proceedings of the National Academy of Sciences, USA 94 (1997): 3519–3523.

Green, A.E., & R.F. Alison, "Recombination between viral RNA and transgenic plant transcripts," *Science* 263 (1994): 1423–1425.

Hileman, B., "Views differ sharply over benefits, risks of agricultural biotechnology," *Chemical and Engineering News,* August 21, 1995.

Mead, P.S., Slutsker, L., Dietz, V., et al.. "Food-related illness and death in the United States," *Emerg. Infect. Dis.* 5 (1999): 607–25.

Mississippi State University Cooperative Extension Service, *Broiler Litter as a Feed or Fertilizer in Livestock Operations,* 1998.

MMWR Weekly Report, April 13, 2007, 56(14): 336–339.

Moore, Oliver, "U.S. strain of *E. coli* strikes Canadian," *The Globe and Mail* (Toronto), September 26, 2006, A15.

National Heart, Lung, and Blood Institute, *Clinical Guidelines on the Identification, Evaluation, and Treatment of Overweight and Obesity in Adults,"* Department of Health and Human Services, National Institutes of Health, 1998, NIH Publication no. 98–4083.

National Task Force on Prevention and Treatment of Obesity, "Overweight, obesity, and health risk," *Archives of Internal Medicine,* 160(7) (2000): 898–904.

New England Journal of Medicine, 345, no. 16 (2001): 1155–1160.

New York Times, "You are what you grow," April 22, 2007, at http://www.nytimes.com/2007/04/22/magazine.

Partnership for Healthy Weight Management, *Weight Loss:Finding a Weight Loss Program That Works for You, 2000,* at www.consumer.gov/weightloss/brochures.htm.

Partnership for Healthy Weight Management, *Setting Goals for Healthy Weight Loss*, 1999, at www.consumer.gov/weightloss/brochures.htm.

Pollan, Michael, *The Omnivore's Dilemma: A Natural History of Four Meals,* (New York: Penguin, 2006).

President's Council on Physical Fitness and Sports, Department of Health and Human Services, *Exercise and Weight Control,* at www.fitness.gov/Reading_Room/reading_room.html.

Shaik, S., Helmers, G., & Atwood, J., "The evolution of farm programs and their contribution to agricultural land value," *American Journal of Agricultural Economics,* vol. 87, No. 5 (2005): 1190–1197.

Schlosser, Eric, *Fast Food Nation—The Dark Side of the All-American Meal* (Portland: Houghton Mifflin, 2001).

Schnepf, Randy, & Womach, Jasper. *Potential Challenges to US Farm Subsidies in the WTO,* CRS Report for Congress RL336697 (Washington, DC: Congressional Research Service, Oct. 25, 2006).

USAID.gov/about_usaid/presidential_initiative/endhunger.html.

U.S. Department of Agriculture and U.S. Department of Health and Human Services, *Dietary Guidelines for Americans.* 2000.

USDA Proposal for the 2007 Farm Bill, at www.usda.gov/ documents/07finalfbp.pdf.

USDA, "Summary XIII: Socially Disadvantaged Producers," at www.usda.gov/documents/ 07sumdisadvantagedsupport.pdf.

Weise, Elizabeth, "Poison pet food woes seem to hit cats harder," *USA Today,* May 8, 2007.

World Health Organization, *World Health Report, Life in the 21st century: A Vision for All.* (Geneva: World Health Organization, 1998) 132.

Chapter

6

ENVIRONMENTAL HEALTH

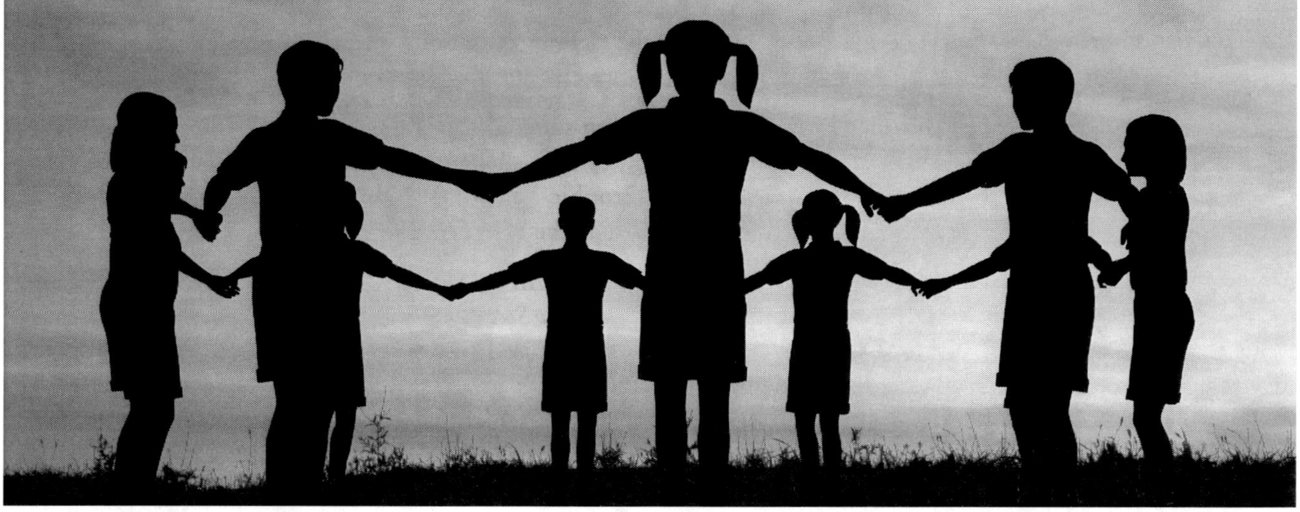

We do not inherit the earth from our ancestors; we borrow it from our children.

—Native American Proverb

As human beings, we are all part of the environment, and the ways in which we interact with our environment greatly influences the quality of our lives. **Environmental health** is all of the physical, chemical, biological, social, and psychosocial factors in the environment. It also refers to the theories and practices involved in assessing, correcting, controlling, and preventing factors in the environment that can potentially adversely affect the health of present and future generations.

Environmental hazards are dangers in the environment. They might be biological, chemical, physical, psychological, or sociological dangers. The exploitation of natural resources, such as the destruction of forests, the building of new land, and the contamination of water, have caused alarming changes in the environment in recent decades, often harming the most vulnerable people in the world, who depend on natural resources for survival.

The physical environment also has a significant impact on people's health behaviors. One study by the World Health Organization (WHO) estimated that about 35% of deaths caused by cancer are a result of lifestyle and environmental factors, including the following:

- being overweight and obese,
- having low fruit and vegetable intake,
- lack of physical activity,
- smoking,
- using alcohol in excess,
- having unsafe sex, and
- urban air pollution.

Did you know?

- More than 2.4 billion people worldwide do no [illegible] e access to proper sanitation facilities, and 1 billion people do not have access to safe drinking water.
- An estimated 2 million children die every year- [illegible] 00 a day—from preventable infections that are spread by contaminated water or unsafe sanitation faciliti[illegible]
- Approximately 2 billion of the world's poorest [illegible] do not have regular access to energy supplies for heating and cooking, which forces them to clear tree [illegible] n rain forests and other valuable forests for firewood or to burn heavily polluting fuels, such as kerosene, [illegible] are harmful to human health.
- The disproportionately high energy consumption [illegible] richest countries has caused greenhouse gas emissions to spike, which could ultimately result in potentia[illegible] ire changes in Earth's climates.
- Climate changes are expected to have the greatest e[illegible] on some of the poorest regions in the world. Possible consequences of climate changes include the altera[illegible] of rainfall patterns that will impact agriculture, the spreading of diseases such as malaria, and more cat[illegible] phic and frequent extreme weather events that the people of poor countries are ill equipped to handle, s[illegible] s the tsunami that swept over Thailand in 2004.

Any time that humans change the environment, there pot[illegible] ly will be repercussions related to health, including the risk of increased incidences of diseases. In the book *Coll[illegible] ow Societies Choose to Fail or Succeed*, Jared Diamond presents many examples of cultures that died out because [illegible] refused to change their traditional habits of how they interacted with the environment. For example, the R[illegible] i, a group of people who lived on a Polynesian island, were obsessed with building large stone figures calle[illegible] i, which they moved using wooden ramps made from trees. The Rapanui eventually clear-cut the entire islar[illegible] ich led to the extinction of animals and plants, starvation, and social chaos.

The consequences of international trade, economic policies, a[illegible] control of land by governments or the most powerful have caused immense poverty, hunger, and less access [illegible] among the less powerful. The United States consumes far more energy and raw materials per person than an[illegible] country on Earth. The richest 20% of people in the highest-income countries account for 86% of total exper[illegible] for private consumption worldwide, while the poorest 20% of people account for just 1.3%.

Some of the major factors that contribute to a worsening of [illegible] mental hazards include the growth of urbanization, industrialization, populations, and the production c[illegible] ble products and containers.

Many human activities generate wastes and residues as by-product[illegible] y-products include the following:

1. human body wastes;
2. trash and garbage from food and other packages;
3. organic wastes, such as grass and shrub clippings;
4. construction and manufacturing wastes, such as scrap wood, meta[illegible] ated water, chemical solvents, heat, and noise;
5. transportation wastes, such as carbon monoxide, nitrous oxides, hyd[illegible] other pollutants, and used motor oil; and
6. energy-production wastes, including wastes from mining, electrical powe[illegible] on (combustion of coal), nuclear power plants (whose wastes are radioactive), and the manufacture o[illegible]

Overpopulation

The health of the environment would not be an issue if there were unlimited land, wat[illegible] sources on Earth. However, this is not the case. The human population on Earth continues to grow and is [illegible] ted to be greater than 6 billion people, all of whom must share the same piece of the resources pie but wi[illegible] ller and smaller portions. Overpopulation has created other problems, such as the potential to cause health epidemics; as people meet more and more people, the more and different types of contagious germs and viruses they can pick up and pass along to others. Overpopulation also creates the problems of sanitation and pollution, which can also contribute to health epidemics. However, overpopulation is just one of the factors in the worsening conditions of the environment. Other factors include how and where people choose to live and how they produce, consume, and often waste Earth's resources.

Human behaviors that impact the environment:

- agricultural burning,
- over-consumption of resources,
- failure to recycle,
- improper disposal of toxic wastes,
- improper disposal of human wastes,
- improper disposal of trash,
- overuse and misuse of pesticides,
- overcrowding,
- depletion of soils by over-farming,
- removal of vegetation,
- urban sprawl,
- over-fishing,
- removal of trees without replanting,
- inefficient use of fuels,
- urbanizing farmland,
- urban growth where water is scarce,
- eating and mass producing meat,
- wars, and
- environmental disasters caused by humans.

A Brief History of Environmental Disasters:

9/11 Dust

The destruction of the World Trade Center (WTC) on September 11 of 2001 was the largest environmental disaster that New York City had ever experienced. Amid all the rubble, asbestos was of great concern not only to government agencies in New York City, but also to the public. Asbestos form the destruction of the two towers settled at Ground Zero and in nearby apartments, office buildings, and schools.

Facts about Asbestos:

- It is a fibrous form of mineral silicates.
- Its fibers can lodge in the lungs, abdomen, brain, and heart of humans.
- It can cause mesothelioma, a fatal cancer more painful and devastating even than AIDS.
- It can cause asbestosis, which causes death in humans by cutting off their blood supply.

- It can lay dormant in the lungs for years and then suddenly become active (almost like a ticking time bomb inside the lungs).
- Large but unknown amounts of asbestos are contained within the structures of older commercial and residential buildings.

Fallout from 9/11:

- Some scientists have claimed that the Environmental Protection Agency and other government agencies mislead the public about the asbestos fallout.
- Thousands of workers and visitors were exposed to asbestos and now have the cough characteristic of such exposure.
- Police officers, firefighters, and other first responders became ill with respiratory problems including asthma, cancer (leukemia), and kidney and heart problems. A study released by the Mount Sinai Medical Center in 2004 found that three fourth of them had contracted diseases.

In the largest health study ever conducted by doctors at Mount Sinai Medical Center, findings indicate that the negative impacts on the health of the rescue and recovery efforts of the thousands of workers who labored at Ground Zero have been more widespread and persistent than had previously been thought, and that these negative impacts are likely to linger far into the future. An estimated 70% of the nearly 10,000 workers who were tested at Mount Sinai between 2002 to 2004 reported that they had newly developed or substantially worsened respiratory problems while or after working at Ground Zero. The study is among the first to show that many respiratory problems, such as sinusitis and asthma, as well as gastrointestinal problems related to these problems that were first reported by those who worked at Ground Zero persisted or worsened in the years after 9/11. The study reported that the toxic nature of the dust resulting from the collapse of the towers would remain a serious health issue in the city for years to come. The dust contained tiny shards of glass, which could become lodged in the lungs, as well as a mixture of toxic and carcinogenic substances, including asbestos and dioxin, that could all have the potential for causing cancer decades into the future.

As the health problems caused by 9/11 continue to expand, concern is also growing about the cost of health care for the responders and workers, especially the 40% who either did not have health insurance at the time or who lost the health care coverage provided by their employers after they became too ill to continue working.

Chernobyl

On April 26, 1986, testing was being conducted in a nuclear reactor of the Chernobyl nuclear power plant in Ukraine. The plant was located just 80 miles from Kiev, the capital of Ukraine. Both errors in the design of the reactor and errors in judgment of the personnel working at the nuclear power plant caused the cooling water to boil. This disastrous condition created reactor stress that caused energy production to increase to ten times the normal level. Temperatures inside the reactor reached more than 2,000 °C, causing the fuel rods to melt and the cooling water to continue to boil. The extreme pressures that built up in the cooling water pipes caused them to crack, which, in turn, allowed steam to escape from the power plant.

In the middle of the night, the steam that had escaped caused a massive explosion, blowing the roof off the building, igniting a major fire, and forming a huge toxic cloud in the atmosphere that contained an estimated 185 to 250 million curies of radioactive material. The fire and the explosion instantly killed 31 people. The next day, more than 135,000 people were evacuated from within a 30-kilometer radius of the power plant, an area that the government called the special zone. Because the high levels of radioactivity that had escaped from the nuclear reactor were expected to exist in that area for centuries to come, the evacuation of the special zone was permanent. In the meantime, winds blew the huge radioactive cloud north and northwest, and it soon covered a large portion of Europe—even reaching the Netherlands—causing governments to prohibit consumption of fresh fruits and vegetables.

Many scientists have tried to estimate the number of victims that suffered from symptoms caused by radiation from the Chernobyl accident; however, there is still no reliable data. The WHO reported that about 800,000 people worked to extinguish the, restore the reactor, and clean up pollutants in the first year after the accident. People who had lived in the area near Chernobyl at the time of the accident suffered from a variety of health problems. Immediately after the accident, hundreds of people were diagnosed with radiation sickness. In addition, there was a dramatic increase in the number of cases of thyroid cancer and leukaemia, especially in nearby Belarus. Children suffered from birth defects that caused cancer and heart diseases. The combination of all the health problems related to the Chernobyl accident and the fear of death from radiation caused mental illness in many children, and suicide rates increased by 1,000% in the areas nearby.

Three Mile Island

On March 28, 1979, the cooling system of a reactor at the Three Mile Island nuclear power plant near Harrisburg, Pennsylvania, failed. The cooling water drained away from the reactor instead of over it, with the result of a partial meltdown of the reactor core. This caused a release into the atmosphere of approximately one-thousandth the amount of radiation as was released during the Chernobyl explosion.

Studies have indicated that the radiation from the Three Mile Island nuclear reactor contributed to premature deaths, the development of cancers, and birth defects of people who lived in the area at the time of the nuclear meltdown. Dairy farmers also reported that many of their animals had died because of the accident.

Love Canal

By 1920, the Hooker Chemical plant had turned an area in Niagara Falls into a chemical disposal site. A nearby city bought the dumpsite for one dollar with the intention of using it for urban expansion. Blocks of homes and a school were subsequently built, and the neighbourhood was named Love Canal.

Children who lived in the neighbourhood often became ill, and no one knew why. Residents of Love Canal regularly experienced miscarriages and birth defects. When research was conducted, more than 130 pounds of the highly toxic carcinogenic TCDD, a form of dioxin, was discovered in Love Canal. In addition, the total of 20,000 tons of waste that was present in the landfill appeared to contain more than 248 different types of chemicals. However, none of the chemicals were removed from the dumpsite. Instead, the dumpsite was sealed, and the surrounding area was cleaned up and declared safe. Today, the Love Canal dumpsite is known as the first and one of the most disastrous human-caused environmental events of the twentieth century.

The Exxon Valdez

In 1989, the oil-tanker ship *Exxon Valdez* spilled more than 30 million gallons of crude oil into Prince William Sound, just off the coast of Alaska. The spill created a huge oil slick that settled on top of the water. Despite intensive cleanup efforts, the oil spill killed an estimated 250,000 seabirds, 2,800 sea otters, 250 bald eagles, and 22 killer whales. Wildlife biologists and medical researchers now know that particular components of the oil, called polycyclic aromatic hydrocarbons, are deadly. These components can work their way through air, water, soil, and food. They can cause reproduction difficulties, genetic damage, central nervous system problems and respiratory problems, and cancer. Exxon Mobil, the owner of the *Exxon Valdez,* paid approximately 3.5 billion dollars in fines and cleanup costs associated with the oil spill.

Newton Creek

Exxon Mobil is responsible for another environmental disaster, an underground oil spill and leakage into Newtown Creek in New York City. Newton Creek remains one of the nation's most polluted waterways, affecting the health of people in the city. To date, an estimated 17 million gallons of oil have leaked into the creek. The leakage amounts to approximately 6 million gallons more than was spilled by the *Exxon Valdez* in 1989 and remains the largest underground oil spill in U.S. history.

In Greenpoint, a community in Brooklyn that borders the Newton Creek, residents complained about strong petroleum odors and experienced the worst of the spill. Neighborhoods in Queens, including Long Island City, West Maspeth, and Sunnyside, also border the creek. Riverkeeper, an environmental advocacy group dedicated to protecting the ecological integrity of the Hudson River, has warned that the Newtown Creek spill and leakage pose a serious threat to the health of the people who live near the banks of the creek in both Queens and Brooklyn.

New York State Attorney General Andrew Cuomo stated, in reference to the spill and the company's record-shattering profits of $39.5 billion in 2006, "Exxon Mobil has proven itself far less than a model corporate citizen, placing its greed for windfall profits over public safety and the well-being of the environment."

The Gulf War

In August of 1990, Iraqi forces invaded Kuwait, igniting the Gulf War and resulting in two major environmental disasters. The first incident was an oil spill about 10 miles off the shore of Kuwait caused by the dumping of oil from several tankers and the opening of the valves of an offshore terminal. The second incident involved the burning of 650 oil wells in Kuwait. An estimated one million tons of crude oil was lost, making this the largest oil spill in history. In the spring of 1991, as many as 500 oil wells were still burning, and the last one was not extinguished until November.

The oil spills of the Gulf War considerably damaged the environment of the Persian Gulf. Within several months of the spills, the tainted water killed 20,000 seabirds and caused serious damage to marine flora and fauna. The fires in the oil wells released huge amounts of soot and toxic fumes into the atmosphere and might have had an impact on local weather patterns.

Global Warming

Many scientists predict that global warming could lead to a number of environmental problems, including drought, famine, wildfires, a rise in sea level, outbreaks of disease, and numerous environmental refugees.

Did you know?

- Of the hottest 20 years on record, 9 have occurred since 1980.
- The number of category 4 and 5 hurricanes worldwide has nearly doubled over the past 30 years.
- Fatal heat waves are becoming more frequent: At least 179 people died in the heat wave of 2006, and about 52,000 people died in the heat wave that struck Europe in 2003.
- One-third of all amphibian species are at risk of extinction because global warming.
- Entire villages are being relocated in Alaska because the sea ice can no longer support them.

Global warming is the gradual increase in Earth's temperature. The **ozone layer**, part of Earth's stratosphere, protects the planet from the sun's UVB radiation. In the 1970s, researchers discovered that chlorofluorocarbons (CFCs) were contributing to the rapid depletion of the ozone layer. Earth's average surface temperature has risen by 1°F in the past century, with an accelerated increase over the past two decades. Recently, scientists have discovered the first unequivocal link between the emission of human-made greenhouse gases and the dramatic heating of the oceans on Earth. They have explained a strong correlation between the rise in ocean temperatures over the past 40 years and the pollution of the atmosphere. These scientists have predicted that sea levels around the world could rise by more than 20 feet, with significant loss of shelf ice in Greenland and Antarctica, which would devastate coastal areas around the world. Other warnings include increased frequency and intensity of heat waves, and more frequent droughts and wildfires. Some scientists even believe that by 2050, the Arctic Ocean might have no ice during the summer by 2050, and that more than one million species worldwide could become extinct as a result of global warming.

Greenhouse gases include carbon dioxide, chlorofluorocarbons (CFCs), ground-level ozone, nitrous oxide, and methane. These substances form a layer of gases that allows heat from the sun to pass through the atmosphere to Earth but traps the heat as it rises from Earth's surface.

CFC, or chlorofluorocarbons, is the collective name for compounds made of carbon, fluorine, chlorine, and hydrogen. Because they have stable, harmless and noncombustible properties, these compounds are widely used in everyday products, such as coolants for air conditioners, cleaning agents for electronic components, and foaming agents for the manufacture of insulating materials.

Carbon dioxide and other gases naturally warm the surface of Earth by trapping heat from the sun in the atmosphere. The burning of fossil fuels, such as coal, natural gas, and oil, and the clearing of forests has dramatically increased the amount of carbon dioxide in Earth's atmosphere. As a result, global temperatures are rising, glaciers are melting, polar bears are drowning, plants and animals are being forced to leave their habitats, and the frequency of severe storms and droughts is increasing.

Global warming is largely caused by pollution, which is caused by generating and using energy, including electricity from power plants, gasoline in the tanks of cars and trucks, and industrial consumption of coal, oil, and natural gas. Government handouts to big energy companies are responsible for the burning of ever more coal, oil, and natural gas. The problem of global warming requires multiple solutions, including strong governmental regulations and the effective enforcement of such regulations.

As mentioned earlier, Earth's climate has warmed by about 1° F since 1900. Scientists have shown that at least 279 species of plants and animals have responded to this level of global warming by moving closer to the poles. Most regions of the Arctic have experienced a rise in temperature of 4 to 7°F in the past 50 years. These changes are threatening the lives of animals such as polar bears, which live and hunt on the sea ice. Over the past 15 years, polar bears have experienced about a 15% decline in the number of offspring and a similar decrease in weight. If the Arctic sea ice begins to melt completely during the summer by 2050, as some scientists predict, polar bears as a species will have little chance of surviving.

Corals are in danger as well. Not only are coral reefs a beautiful and essential part of the environment, but they also provide protection to coastal areas against storm surges and tsunamis. Some coral species are facing the greatest threat to their survival in 500,000 years. According to a report for the Pew Center on Global Climate Change, one-fourth of the world's coral reefs have already been destroyed. Another study, one by the IUCN-World Conservation Union, warns that half of the existing corals on Earth could be eliminated by the year 2045, when average temperatures are predicted to be as much as 3°F higher than they currently are.

Is New York due for a hurricane?

The nation's largest city is due for a major hurricane, according to Nicholas Coch, Professor of Geology at Queens College and a hurricane expert. Coch predicts that such a hurricane has the potential to create catastrophic effects on New York City. It would wreak havoc on buildings and infrastructures, in addition to forcing the evacuation of an estimated 3 million people, which is more than six times the population of New Orleans before Hurricane Katrina struck. A Category 3 hurricane striking New York City would have the effects of a Category 4 hurricane along the coasts in the South. A major hurricane hitting New York could produce a storm surge of up to 30 feet high, causing flooding in all five boroughs and the closing of airports and highways, not to mention massive traffic jams. The lower Manhattan flood zone for a hurricane making landfall just south of the city includes Wall Street, police headquarters, and the World Trade Center site. City Hall, which is located on higher ground and is more toward the middle of Manhattan, could become a small island as the East River and the Hudson River converge to the south.

Air Pollution

Air pollution is the contamination of the air by substances in amounts great enough to affect human safety, health, and comfort. Major sources of outdoor air pollution include emissions given off by transportation vehicles, electric power plants fueled by oil and coal, and industries.

Acid rain is the depositing on Earth's surface of sulfuric and nitrous acids absorbed from the atmosphere during the formation of rain droplets. Acid rain can damage vegetation as well as the ecosystems of lakes, rivers, and streams.

The ozone layer, as described earlier, plays an important role in protecting life on Earth by absorbing harmful ultraviolet radiation (UVB) from the sun. The ozone layer's depletion is global. A large ozone hole has been observed in the Antarctic Circle. Destruction of the ozone allows greater amount of harmful ultraviolet radiation (UVB) to reach earth's surface, which can result in increased cases of skin cancer and visual health concerns, such as cataracts.

Photochemical smog is a secondary air pollutant that is created when primary pollutants react with sunlight and atmospheric oxygen. Denver, Los Angeles, Phoenix, and Salt Lake City are among the cities in the United States that experience the highest levels of photochemical smog.

Air pollutants also exist indoors. These pollutants are gases or particles of matter inside buildings and are harmful to human health. Some examples of indoor air pollution include asbestos, biogenic pollutants, combustion by-products, formaldehyde, radon, tobacco smoke, and volatile organic compounds.

Health Effects of Global Environmental Change

Environmental Change	Health Effects
Ozone depletion	Skin cancer, cataracts
Temperature extremes	Heat stroke, malaria, malnutrition
Decreased precipitation resulting in droughts	Malnutrition, asthma, allergies, respiratory diseases
Increased frequency of floods and hurricanes diseases	Cholera, diarrheal malnutrition, death

Lead Poisoning

Lead is a harmful toxin and the major environmental hazard for children. Lead is a naturally occurring element that is used in the manufacture of many industrial and household products. Power plants and other industrial facilities emit lead into the air, where it eventually settles into the soil and dust. This lead is then brought into homes or ingested by children as they play outdoors and put their hands in their mouths. Very young children are particularly at risk of lead poisoning by putting pieces of lead paint peeling from walls into their mouths. Recent investigations have revealed that many toys, especially those made in China, are contaminated with lead. Health problems associated with lead include anemia, birth defects, and bone, neurological, and damage. For children, even small amounts of lead have been shown to lower IQ levels.

Solutions for the prevention of lead poisoning include education, regulation of the use of lead, and individual responsibility for knowing what materials contain lead and avoiding using or coming in contact with them.

Prevention of lead poisoning includes the following

- **Avoid direct contact with soil,** especially if you live in an urban area or near a highway.
- **Wash your hands as soon as you get home from work.**
- **Take your shoes off at the door** to avoid bringing contaminated soil into the home.
- **Vacuum carpets frequently** using an HEPA vacuum cleaner. Use a damp rag frequently to clean painted wooden windowsills, moldings, and floors.
- **Check for peeling or flaking paint**, especially if your home was built before 1978. Have the paint tested by a professional service or with a home testing kit.
- **Test imported dishware or pottery** before cooking or serving food in it. Lead paints and glazes are still used outside the United States and Europe. Lead-contaminated dishes and pottery—particularly from Mexico and China—have recently been found in stores in the United States.
- **Let tap water run for a few minutes** before you drink it to make sure that any water that has been standing in the pipes has run through.
- **Use charcoal filters for water, including filters for pitchers.**

Malaria is a disease caused by mosquitoes and transmitted from person to person. It kills between one and two million people annually, mainly in tropical parts of Africa, and debilitates as many as 400 million others. Scientists believe that climate is the major factor in the spread of malaria, because mosquitoes live in warm, humid environments. In warm regions of the world other than Africa, methods of repelling and killing mosquitoes, including netting and mass-spraying of pesticides, are largely responsible for limiting the incidences of malaria.

Asthma is a chronic, inflammatory lung disease whose symptoms include recurring episodes of breathlessness, wheezing, coughing, and chest tightness. These episodes are known as exacerbations or attacks. National data indicate that the number of children who have asthma in the United States has more than doubled in the past 15 years. Asthma is a growing concern especially for African-American and Latino children who live in inner-cities. Estimates indicate that one out of four African American children living in New York City has asthma. African-American children age 4 and younger are six times as likely as white children of similar ages to die from asthma, and even those who escape death are hospitalized more often than are white children. In other developed countries, the number of children who are diagnosed with asthma has also increased significantly. Most scientists attribute this rise in the incidence of childhood asthma on air pollution. The environment is a major factor in the onset and severity of asthma.

Chemicals and biological agents that increase the risk of an asthma attack include the following:

- Second-hand smoke from cigarettes, especially in indoor environments, brings on asthma attacks in many people who are sensitive, and it may be a cause the development of asthma in younger children.
- Allergens produced by dust mites, cockroaches, mold, and pets in homes can trigger wheezing and other symptoms of asthma in those who are allergic to them.
- Exposure to ozone or diesel exhaust exacerbates the effects of allergies on asthma, but about 99% of U.S. school buses run on diesel fuel.

Other factors that contribute to the development and exacerbation of asthma include living in poor housing conditions, living in urban areas near high-traffic roads, and lack of access to adequate medical care.

What do hamburgers have to do with the environment?

It is widely known that industrial farms illegally dump millions of tons of untreated fecal and toxic waste onto land and into water. This type of farming has contaminated numerous bodies of water, killed billions of fish and other organisms, sickened consumers, and subjected millions of animals to cruel treatment.

Cattle emit huge volumes of methane, a gas that is 23 times more efficient in trapping heat than carbon dioxide is. The manure of cattle bred for meat is the source of two-thirds of human-caused nitrous oxide, a greenhouse gas that is 300 times as potent as carbon dioxide. The farming of corn, soybeans, and hay for livestock feed accounts for about half of all fertilizers used in the United States, and generates large amounts of nitrous oxide. In Brazil, thousands of acres of rain forests are being cut down to clear the land for pastures and fields in which to grow animal feed.

One solution that individuals can participate in to reduce global environmental changes is to eat less meat and more whole foods, such as beans, nuts, fruits and vegetables. Such a diet also reduces the risk of obesity, diabetes, and heart disease.

Water

Water is a necessity for all forms of life, yet access to safe and clean drinking water is a huge concern for many people around the world. Only about 3% of the water on Earth is freshwater, and two-thirds of that water is unavailable in glaciers. The main sources of freshwater are rainwater; surface water from streams, lakes, and rivers; and groundwater.

A person can survive for a month or longer without food but only for about three days without water. Thousands of chemicals that are used in industrial processes, as well as lead, sewage, and gasoline have been found in tap water in the United States. It is safest to drink charcoal-filtered water, water that has been boiled (which still does not eliminate lead), or bottled spring water.

All tap water has chemicals added to it, specifically chlorine and fluoride. Some scientists believe that these chemicals cause high levels of toxicity, which can scar the arteries. Fluoride affects the thyroid gland. The United States has the highest levels of fluoride in tap water in the world and also the highest obesity rate. Fluoride has been linked to depression and physical problems, some related to thyroid activity and possibly even obesity. Chlorine is a poison, and high doses of it kills living organisms.

The U.S. Environmental Protection Agency (EPA) routinely assures the public that nearly 100% of community water systems meet clean drinking water standards. However, in a test by the Environmental Working Group of tap water from a variety of cities, the group found 119 "normal" chemicals (those for which the EPA allows in water but has set limits) and another 141 chemicals that are completely unregulated.

Water quality in the United States is threatened by four conditions:

1. Population growth;
2. Growth of the chemical industry;
3. Environmental mismanagement, including irresponsible disposal of wastes; and
4. Reckless land-use practices.

Chemical water pollution typically occurs for the following reasons:

- Chemicals were dumped into the water intentionally;
- Chemicals seeped into groundwater, streams, or rivers through leaky pipes or storage tanks;
- Chemicals contaminated bodies of water as a result of industrial accidents; and
- Pollution was cycled from polluted air through rainwater; and
- Chemicals were leached out of contaminated soil.

The types of chemical contamination described above are called **point sources** of water pollution. **Non-point-sources** are sources that cause pollution of water secondhand, as pesticide runoff from farm fields and lawns, as well as runoff of automotive fluids and other chemicals from roads, parking lots, driveways, and other surfaces, flow into bodies of water or seep into groundwater.

Biological hazards include organisms that are harmful to humans, such as water-borne diseases that are transmitted through drinking water. Examples of biological hazards include the polio virus, the hepatitis A virus, salmonella, shigella, cholera, amoebic dysentery, and cryptosporidium. These disease–causing organisms are transported into water from feces, and they can cause illnesses in people who drink or cook with this untreated, contaminated water.

Pesticides are chemicals that are manufactured to destroy pests. Pesticides include herbicides and insecticides. The misuse or overuse of pesticides can result in illness and even death in humans.

The best-known case of pesticide pollution in the United States occurred in the 1960s,when the insecticide DDT was found to have polluted waterways, which then contaminated fish and poisoned animals that ate the fish. DDT was banned from agricultural use in the United States in 1972 and shortly thereafter was banned worldwide at the Stockholm Convention after concerns were raised, largely as a result of the research and efforts of biologist Rachael Carson, over its effects on the environment, and on animal and human health. DDT was alleged to be a liver and breast carcinogen, and women who were exposed to the pesticide were found to have higher than normal rates of infertility. However, DDT it is still used in some developing countries to destroy malaria-carrying mosquitoes. Many Americans continue to be exposed to DDT through produce that was grown in tropical countries, as well as through fish caught in some U.S. waters.

In terms of general human health, pesticides can have the following effects:

- damage the nervous system,
- cause liver damage,

- damage DNA and cause a variety of cancers, and
- cause reproductive and endocrine damage.

Intersex fish

Many of the chemicals that are dumped into waterways in the United States disrupt hormones. These chemicals cause interrupted sexual development in fish in water with high hormone concentrations; that is, female fish begin to exhibit male fish characteristics and vice versa.

Other effects on fish include thyroid system disorders, the inability to breed, weakened immune responses, and abnormal mating and other behaviors. In humans, hormone disruptors lead to weakened immune functions, mental impairments, increases in the incidences of infertility, and increases in the development of some types of cancers.

What Can You Do to Help the Environment?

With less than 5% of the world's population, the United States produces between one-fifth and one-fourth of the world's greenhouse-gas emissions. In addition, more than 100 million trees are cut down every year to produce junk mail, not to mention the 28 billion gallons of water that are used for this purpose. The energy resources annually used to produce and dispose of junk mail exceeds the amount used to power 2.8 million cars.

Conserve Energy

People can conserve energy by driving hybrid cars, using public transportation, installing solar panels in their homes, and using fluorescent light bulbs. People can also lobby companies to stop sending unsolicited junk mail and catalogues, which contribute to the destruction of the rain forests.

Reduce Pollution

Individuals and groups can help to develop national strategies and policies to address air pollution. They also can support policies that encourage the use of renewable resources, and use and support alternative methods of transportation. Most experts agree that alternative methods of transportation are necessary to reduce air pollution significantly.

Stop the Destruction of Rain Forests

The most recent estimates indicate that approximately 150,000 square kilometers of tropical rain forests, roughly equal to the size of England and Wales combined, is destroyed every year. Rain forests are valuable for a variety of reasons. First, they continuously recycle carbon dioxide into oxygen. In fact, more than 20% of the world's oxygen is produced in the Amazon Rain Forest, followed by the Congo of Central Africa, which is the second-largest rain forest on Earth. Millions of people depend on the rain forests for their survival, and obtain food, medicine, and shelter there. The rain forests are also essential in the regulation of local and global climates. Thus, it is important that people make every effort to stop the destruction of the rain forests.

Rain forests are destroyed because they are

- rich in minerals, including oil, gold, aluminum, iron, and cobalt;
- used for seismic testing for oil;
- used by the logging industry;
- used for the cutting of tracks and routes for oil pipelines;
- used for commercial and subsistence farming;
- used by huge plantations of rubber trees, within which bananas, soy beans, and oil palms are also grown
- used for the production of paper

Scientists estimate that nearly half of the world's species of plants, animals, and microorganisms will be destroyed or threatened over the next several decades as a result of rain forest destruction. As their homelands continue to be destroyed by deforestation, indigenous rain forest peoples are also disappearing. Five hundred years ago, an estimated 10 million Native Americans lived in the Amazonian Rain Forest, while today, there are less than 200,000. If deforestation continues at current rates, scientists estimate that between 80 and 90% of the tropical rain forests' ecosystems could be destroyed by the year 2020.

Simple Ways That You Can Improve Earth's Health

Environmental scientists warn that global warming will affect every person, community, and nation, creating a cycle of events likely to have harmful results. People's choices about where to live, work, and travel, and what to buy have a profound effect on their health and on the health of others around the world. The following are ways in which individuals can make a positive impact on the environment:

- Switch to highly efficient compact fluorescent light bulbs (CFLs) that last for years, use only one-fourth of the energy of regular light bulbs, and actually produce more light.
- Buy a fuel-efficient car, such as a hybrid. Replacing gas-guzzling cars with fuel-efficient ones is by far the most important contribution that an individual can make. Although automakers haven't yet sold enough hybrids in the United States to make them as affordable as they should be, this will change if there is a demand for more hybrids, and less for the gas guzzlers.
- Turn off equipment such as televisions and stereos when they are not in use. The little red standby light means that they are still using power and that means a contribution to global warming.
- Conserve water by turning off the tap while brushing your teeth and by collecting the water used to wash vegetables and salad greens to water houseplants.
- Call 311 to find a disposal location for used car batteries, cell phones, and other hazardous household wastes items.
- Recycle paper, glass, plastics, and other waste.
- Use rechargeable batteries.
- Don't use "throw-away" products such as paper plates and napkins, or plastic knives, forks, and cups, because these contribute to more garbage.
- Celebrate Earth Day by organizing and participating in protests to preserve our land.
- Work to find alternative energy sources.
- Elect officials who fight against corporate polluters, not give them tax breaks.

References

Amoco Cadiz, http://greennature.com/article219.html.

Arctic Climate Impact Assessment, *Impacts of a Warming Arctic* (Cambridge: Cambridge University Press, 2004). Also quoted in *Time Magazine,* "Vicious Cycles", Missy Adams, March 26, 2006.

Bjerklie, David, "Feeling the Heat," *Time Magazine,* March 26, 2006.

Carson, Rachel, *Silent Spring* (Portland: Mariner Books, 2002).

Chernobyl, at http://www.chernobyl.co.uk/ and the Chernobyl Children's Project International, at http://www.chernobyl-international.com/aboutchernobyl/disaster.asp.

Colborn, T., "Pesticides—How research has succeeded and failed to translate science into policy: Endocrinological effects on wildlife," *Environmental Health Perspectives Supplements* 103 (Suppl 6) (1995): 81–86.

Conin, John, & Kennedy, Robert Jr, *The Riverkeeper: Two Activists Fight to Reclaim Our Environment as a Basic Human Right*, 1st Touchstone ed. (Portland: Scribner,1999).

Columbia University, World Trade Center Environmental Contaminant Database (WTCECD) (New York: Mailman School of Public Health, Columbia University, 2003). Available at http://wtc.hs.columbia .edu/wtc/.

Dejmek J, Selevan, S.G., Benes, I., Solansky, I., & Sram, R.J., "Fetal growth and maternal exposure to particulate matter during pregnancy," *Environ Health Perspect* 107 (1999: 475–480.

Diamond, J., *Collapse: How Societies Choose to Fail or Succeed* (New York: Viking, 2005).

Dodson, R.F., Williams, M.G., Corn, C.J., Brollo, A., & Bianchi, C., "A comparison of asbestos burden in lung parenchma, lymph nodes and plaques," *Ann NY Acad Sci* 643 (1991): 53–60.

Edelman P., Osterloh, J., Pirkle, J., Caudill, S.P., Grainger, J., Jones, R., et al., "Biomonitoring of chemical exposure among New York City firefighters responding to the World Trade Center fire and collapse," *Environ Health Perspect* 111 (2003):1906–1911.

Eilperin, J., "Debate on Climate Shifts to Issue of Irreparable Change," *The Washington Post,* January 29, 2006, A1.

Emanuel, K., "Increasing destructiveness of tropical cyclones over the past 30 years," *Nature* 436 (2005): 686–688.

ENDS, "Pesticides in drinking water linked to breast cancer," ENDS Report 241 (1995): 8–9.

Fairbrother, G., Stuber, J., Galea, S., Fleischman, A.R., & Pfefferbaum, B., "Posttraumatic stress reactions in New York City children after the September 11, 2001, terrorist attacks," *Ambul Pediatrics* 3 (2003): 304–311.

Galea, S., Ahern, J., Resnick, H., Kilpatrick, D., Bucuvalas, M., Gold, J., et al., "Psychological sequelae of the September 11 terrorist attacks in New York City," *N Engl J Med* 346 (2002): 982–987.

Galea, S., Resnick, H., Ahern, J., Gold, J., Bucuvalas, M., Kilpatrick, D., et al., 2002b. "Posttraumatic stress disorder in Manhattan, New York City, after the September 11th terrorist attacks," *J Urban Health* 79 (2002): 340–353.

Gavett, S.H., Haykal-Coates, N., Highfill, J.W., Ledbetter, A.D., Chen, L.C., Cohen, M.D., et al., "World Trade Center fine particulate matter causes respiratory tract hyperresponsiveness in mice," *Environ Health Perspect* 111 (2003): 981–991.

Gibbs, Lois Marie, *Love Canal: The Story Continues,* 20 anniv. ed. (British Columbia: New Society Publishers, 1998).

Gore, Al, *An Inconvenient Truth: The Planetary Emergency of Global Warming and What We Can Do About It* (New York: Rodale Books, 2006).

http://www.nasa.gov.

http://www.pewclimate.org.

http://www.washingtonpost.com/2006/08/03.

http://news.nationalgeographic.com/2006.

http://ww.arctic.noaa.gov.

Institute for Environment and Health, "Environmental oestrogens: Consequences to human health and wildlife," (Leicester: University of Leicester,1995).

Jacobson, S.W., Jacobson, J.L., O'Neill, J.M., Padgett, R.J., Frankowski, J.J., & Bihun, J.T., "Visual expectation and dimensions of infant information processing," Child Dev 63 (1992):711–724.

Kennedy, Robert Jr, *Crimes Against Nature: How George W. Bush and His Corporate Pals Are Plundering the Country and Hijacking Our Democracy* (New York: Harper Perennial, 2005).

Kennedy, Robert Jr, ,"Crimes Against Nature," *Rolling Stone Magazine,* December 11, 2003.

Kogevinas, M., "Human health effects of dioxins: cancer, reproductive and endocrine system effects," *Hum Reprod* 7 (2001): 331–339.

Krabill, W., E. Hanna, P. Huybrechts, W. Abdalati, J. Cappelen, B. Csatho, E. Frefick, S. Manizade, C. Martin, J, Sonntag, R. Swift, R. Thomas, & J. Yungel, "Greenland Ice Sheet: Increased coastal thinning," *Geophysical Research Letters* 31 (2004).

Kelce, W. R., Stone, C. R., Laws, S. C., Gray, L. E., Kemppainen, J. A. & Wilson, E. M., "Persistent DDT metabolite p, p'-DDE is a potent androgen receptor antagonist," *Nature* 375 (1995): 581–585.

Landrigan, P.J., "Health consequences of the 11 September 2001 attacks," *Environ Health Perspect* 109 (2001): A514–A515.

LeBouffant, L., Martin, J.C., Durif, W., & Daniel, H., "Structure and composition of pleural plaque," *IARC Sci Publ* 8 (1973):249–257.

LeBlanc, G. A., "Are environmental sentinels signaling?" *Environ. Health Perspective* 103 (1995): 888–890.

Levin S., Herbert, R., Skloot, G., Szeinuk, J., Teirstein, A., Fischler, D., et al. "Health effects of World Trade Center site workers," *Am J Ind Med* 42 (2001): 545–547.

Lioy, P.J., Weisel, C.P., Millette, J.R., Eisenreich, S., Vallero, D., Offenberg, J., et al.,:Characterization of the dust/smoke aerosol that settled east of the World Trade Center (WTC) in Lower Manhattan after the collapse of the WTC 11 September 2001," *Environ Health Perspect* 110 92002):703–714.

Lippy, B.E., "Safety and health of heavy equipment operators at Ground Zero," *Am J Ind Med* 42 (2002):539–542.

Lomborg, B., *The Skeptical Environmentalist—Measuring the Real State of the World* Cambridge: Cambridge University Press, 1998).

Maynard, R., "Sperm alert," *Living Earth* 188 (995): 8–9.

McKinney, M.L. & Schoch, R.M., *Environmental Science: Systems and Solutions*, 3rd ed. (Sudbury, Massachusetts: Jones and Bartlett, 2003).

Magnani, C., Dalmasso, P., Biggeri, A., Ivaldi, C., Mirabelli, D., & Terracini, B., "Increased risk of malignant mesothelioma of the pleura after residential or domestic exposure to asbestos: a case-control study in Casale Monferrato, Ital,". *Environ Health Perspect* 109 (2001): 915–919.

Malievskaya, E., Rosenberg, N., & Markowitz, S.. "Assessing the health of immigrant workers near Ground Zero: preliminary results of the World Trade Center Day Laborer Medical Monitoring Project," *Am J Ind Med* 42 (2002): 548–549.

McCurdy, T., Glen, G., Smith, L., & Lakkadi, Y., "The national exposure research laboratory's consolidated human activity database," *J Expo Anal Environ Epidemiol* 10(6 Pt 1) (2000): 566–578.

McGee, J.K., Chen, L.C., Cohen, M.D., Chee, G.R., Prophete, C.M., Haykal-Coates, N., et al. Chemical analysis of World Trade Center fine particulate matter for use in toxicological assessment," *Environ Health Perspect* 111 (2003): 972–980.

Nicholson, W.J., & Landrigan, P.J. "Asbestos: A status report," *Curr Issues Public Health* 2 (1996): 118–123.

Nicholson, W.J., Rohl, A.N., Ferrand, E.F., "Asbestos air pollution in New York City," in *Proceedings of the Second International Clean Air Congress,* Englund, H.M, & Beery, W.T., eds. (New York: Academic Press, 1971), 36–139.

NOAA Oil Spill Review, 2003, at http://response.restoration.noaa.gov/oilaids/spilldb.pdf.

Offenberg, J.H., Eisenreich, S.J., Chen, L.C., Cohen, M.D., Chee, G., Prophete, C., et al., "Persistent organic pollutants in the dusts that settled across lower Manhattan after September 11, 2001," *Environ Sci Technol* 37 (2003): 502–508.

Perera, F.P., Whyatt, R.M., Jedrychowski, W., Rauh ,V., Manchester, D., Santella, R.M., et al., "Recent developments in molecular epidemiology: A study of the effects of environmental polycyclic aromatic hydrocarbons on birth outcomes in Poland," *Am J Epidemiol* 147 (1998): 309–314.

Prezant, D.J., Weiden, M., Banauch, G.I., McGuinness, G., Rom, W.N., & Aldrich, T.K. Cough and bronchial responsiveness in firefighters at the World Trade Center site," *N Engl J Med* 347 (2002): 806–815.

Pruss-Ustun A., & Corvalen C., "Preventing disease through healthy environments: Toward an estimate of the environmental burden of disease," (Geneva: World Health Organization, 2006).

Reibman, J., Lin, S., Matte, T., Rogers, L., Hoerning, A., Hwang, S., et al., "Respiratory health of residents near the former World Trade Center: The WTC Residents Respiratory Health Survey" (abstract),. *Am J Respir Crit Care Med* 167 (2003): A335.

Reitze, W.B,, Nicholson, W.J., Holaday, D.A., & Selikoff, I,J., "Application of sprayed inorganic fiber containing asbestos: Occupational health hazards," *Am Ind Hyg Assoc J* 33 (1972):178–191.

Ritz, B., Yu, F., Chapa, G., & Fruin, S., "Effect of air pollution on preterm birth among children born in Southern California between 1989 and 1993," *Epidemiology* 11 (2000): 502–511.

Rom, W.N., Weiden, M., Garcia, R., Yie, T.A., Vathesatogkit, P., Tse, D.B., et al., "Acute eosinophilic pneumonia in a New York City firefighter exposed to World Trade Center dust," *Am J Respir Crit Care Med* 166 (2002): 797–800.

Scanlon, M.D., "World Trade Center cough—A lingering legacy and a cautionary tale," *N Engl J Med* 347 (2002): 840–842.

Schlenger, W.E., Caddell, J.M., Ebert, L., Jordan, B.K., Rourke, K.M., Wilson, D., et al.,"Psychological reactions to terrorist attacks: Findings from the National Study of Americans' Reactions to September 11,"*JAMA* 288 (2002): 581–588.

Sharpe, R. M., "Another DDT connection," *Nature* 375 (1995): 538–539.

Shepherd, P.A., Fagan, J.F., *The Fagan Test of Infant Intelligence* (Cleveland: Infantest Corp., 1987).

Soto, A.M., Sonnenschein, C., Chung, K.L., Fernandez, M.F., Olea, N. & Serrano, F. O.. "The E-SCREEN assay as a tool to identify estrogens: An update on estrogenic environmental pollutants," *Environ. Health Perspe*ct 103 (suppl. 7) (1995): 113–122.

Spadafora, R., "Firefighter safety and health issues at the Word Trade Center site," *Am J Ind Med* 42 (2002): 532–538.

Stuber, J., Fairbrother, G., Galea, S., Pfefferbaum, B., Wilson-Genderson, & M., Vlahov, D., "Determinants of counseling for children in Manhattan after the September 11 attacks," *Psychiatr Serv* 53 (2002): 815–822.

Suzuki, Y., Yuen, S.R., "Asbestos fibers contributing to the induction of human malignant mesothelioma," Annals, *NY Acad Sci* 982 (2002): 160–176.

Taylor, Leslie, *The Healing Power of Rainforest Herbs*, (New York: Square One Publishers, 2004).

Thurston, G., Chen, L.C,. "Risk communication in the aftermath of the World Trade Center disaster," *Am J Ind Med* 42 (2002): 543–544.

Thurston, G., Maciejczyk, P., Lall, R., Hwang, J., & Chen, L.C., "Identification and characterization of World Trade Center Disaster fine particulate matter air pollution at a site in Lower Manhattan following September 11," *Epidemiology* 14 (2003): S87–S88.

U.S. Department of Labor, *Asbestos,*2003, at http://www.osha.gov/SLTC/asbestos/.

U.S. Environmental Protection Agency, *Asbestos Hazard Emergency Response Act (AHERA): Region 2 Compliance,* 1986, at http://www.epa.gov/region02/ahera/ahera.htm.

U.S. Environmental Protection Agency *Exposure and Human Health Evaluation of Airborne Pollution from the World Trade Center Disaster* (External Review Draft), EPA/600/P-2/002A (Washington, D.C.: Environmental Protection Agency, 2002).

U.S. Environmental Protection Agency, at http://www.epa.gov/ncea/wtc.htm.

U.S. Environmental Protection Agency, "Toxicological Effects of Fine Particulate Matter Derived from the Destruction of the World Trade Center," *Fact Sheet: Release of Reports Related to the World Trade Center Disaster. Exposure and Human Health Evaluation of Airborne Pollution from the World Trade Center Disaster* (Washington, D.C.: Environmental Protection Agency, 2003).

U.S. Environmental Protection Agency, *EPA Response to September 11 (Washington, D.C.: Environmental Protection Agency,* 2004), at http://www.epa.gov/wtc/.

Vlahov, D., Galea, S., & Frankel, D., "New York City, 2001: Teaction and response," *J Urban Health* 79 (2002): 2–5.

Vlahov, D., Galea, S., Resnick, H., Ahern, J., Boscarino, J.A., Bucuvalas, M, et al., "Increased use of cigarettes, alcohol, and marijuana among Manhattan, New York, residents after the September 11th terrorist attacks," *Am J Epidemiol* 155 (2002): 988–996.

World Health Organization, at ,www.who.gov/environmentalhealth.

Chapter

7

HEALTH CARE SYSTEM

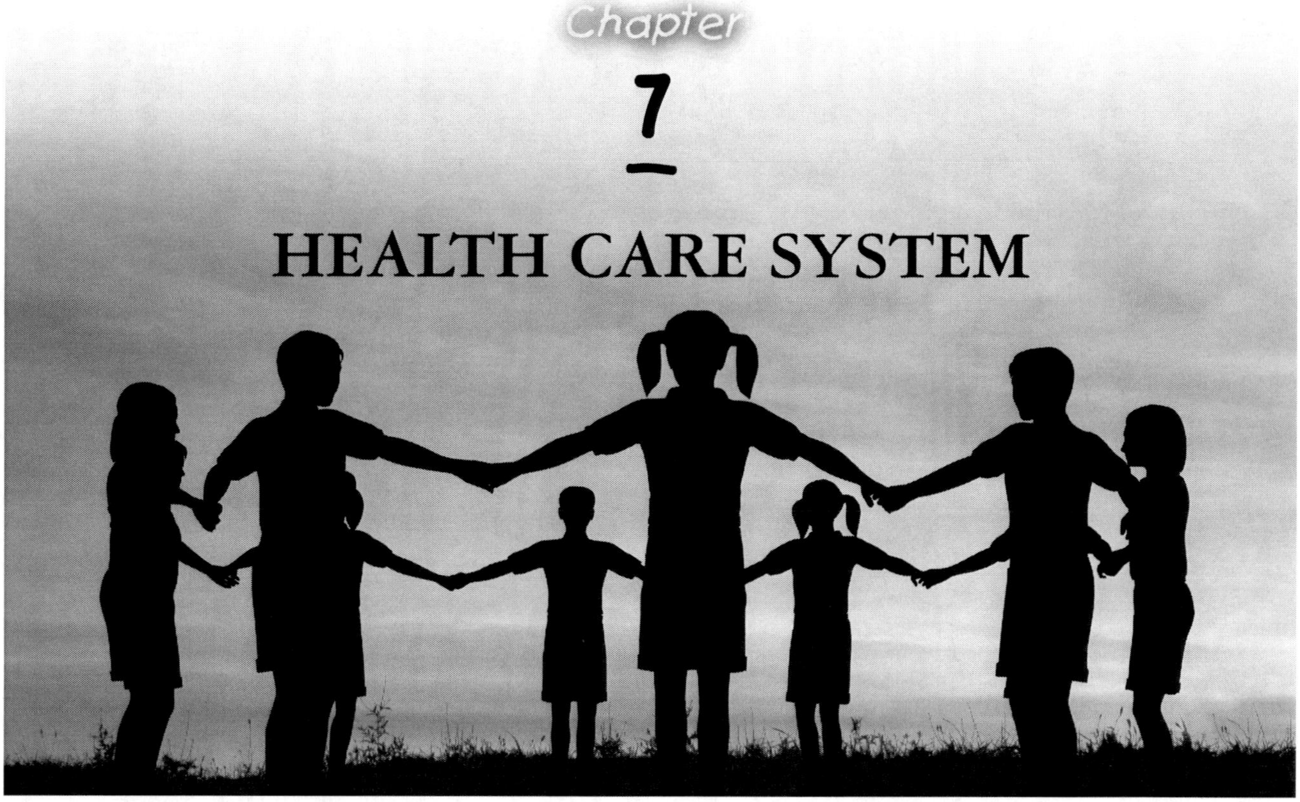

"Of all the forms of inequality, injustice in health care is the most shocking and inhumane."

—Dr. Martin Luther King Jr.

The U.S. health care system is broken, but to fix the system successfully, we must first understand how, why, and where it is broken. The United States spends twice as much money as other developed countries do on health care, yet our health-care system performs poorly in comparison and still leaves about 46 million people without health insurance coverage, including an estimated 9 million children, and millions more with inadequate coverage. The bureaucracy of private insurance companies, including paperwork, consume approximately one-third of every health-care dollar spent. Americans' average life expectancy of age 77 ranks forty-fifth in the world, behind that of Bosnia and Jordan. In addition, the U.S. infant mortality rate is 6.37 per 1,000 live births, higher than that of most developed nations. The World Health Organization (WHO) has ranked the U.S. health care system at thirty-seventh in the world, just behind the war-torn and drug-ravaged country of Columbia.

Many people in this country face major problems with their physical health. Cases of heart disease, diabetes, and obesity are increasing at alarming rates. For the first time in U.S. history, the life expectancy of children today is lower than their parents'.

The cost of health care causes a bankruptcy in the United States every 30 seconds.

A study called "Multinational Comparisons of Health Systems Data," found that, even though the United States spends the most of any country in the world on publicly and privately financed health insurance, Americans have the greatest number of years of life potentially lost as a result of circulatory diseases, respiratory diseases, and diabetes. A 2007 report by the Commonwealth Fund ranked the United States last among other wealthy countries in access to health care, patient safety, efficiency, and equity.

What differences create this disparity between the health care system of the United States and those of other developed countries?

Universal Health Care The United States and South Africa are the only two industrialized countries in the world that do not have a national health-care system that guarantees all citizens access to basic health benefits.

Major issues facing the U.S. health-care system include the following:

- **Health disparities and discrimination:** People who are members of certain ethnic, racial, tribal, and religious minority groups may face health-care discrimination and also experience language and cultural barriers.
- **Costs:** Approximately $2 trillion is spent each year on health care in the United States.
- **Access:** Some communities are underserved or not served at all, with no access to health care.
- **Quality of care and malpractice:** An estimated 44,000 to 98,000 people die every year because of medical errors.
- **Health promotion and disease prevention:** Greater emphasis needs to be placed on these areas of health care.

The United Nations has identified four criteria that are necessary for a successful health-care system. These include the following:

Availability: It is essential that well functioning public health and health-care facilities, services, medicines, and programs are available in sufficient quantity.

Accessibility: Health-care facilities and services must be accessible to all people within a country. Accessibility includes four overlapping factors:

- nondiscrimination,
- physical accessibility,
- affordability, and
- information.

Acceptability: All health-care facilities and services must respect medical ethics, be culturally appropriate, be sensitive to the gender, lifestyle, and age requirements of patients, respect confidentiality, and be designed to improve the health status of patients.

Quality: Health facilities, medicines, and services must be scientifically and medically approved appropriate, and of good quality.

If access to health care is considered a human right, who is considered human enough to have that right?

Access to health care is related to wealth, prestige, education, and power. If health is a human right, then it is a violation of human rights when national and international policies and practices interfere with a person's access to health care. It is unjust that mostly poor people do not have access to even a minimal level of health care.

A lack of health insurance coverage and gaps in such coverage is a problem that has long afflicted lower-income U.S. families. However, this is increasingly becoming a problem that affects many other Americans. The number of people who have no health insurance is increasing, and one of the fastest-growing segments of the national population that is uninsured is people with an income of more than $50,000. In addition, recent college graduates who have not yet found a job often do not have health insurance. Although the lack of health insurance continues to have the highest rate among families with incomes less than $20,000, the rate of people with moderate- and middle-incomes who do not have health insurance is rising, thereby putting not only their health, but also their financial security at risk.

One study of communities in New York City states that the inequitable distribution of health-care services within the city violates state, federal, and international laws that protect people's rights to have access to health care. The study also noted that many neighborhoods with the highest health-care needs, which include disproportionately low-income and minority communities are usually the ones with the fewest health-care resources.

Many poor people are unable to visit doctors for relatively inexpensive preventive care, and thus, when health problems arise, they have no choice but to go to emergency rooms, where the cost of treatment is much higher. An estimated

2 million people in the United States go bankrupt every year as a result of medical debts that they cannot pay. A major study conducted by the Harvard Law School and Medical School indicated that many traditional middle-class families are just one major accident or illness away from economic hardship, bankruptcy, or poverty. According to the study, about half of all personal bankruptcies in the United States are a result, at least partially, of medical debts related to a major accident or illness; about three-fourths of those actually have health insurance at the time of the diagnosis of the illness or accident; and about 68% still have health insurance when they file for bankruptcy .

An estimated 9 million children in the United States do not have health insurance, and many of them are unlikely to receive medical attention for serious injuries or illnesses. In any given year, the death rate for those without health insurance is 25% higher than it is for those who do have health insurance. Poor health and a lack of health insurance is a vicious cycle: because those who are uninsured tend to be less healthy than the general population, they often cannot get better jobs, and therefore they cannot afford health insurance, and when they become ill, they not only infect themselves but also are more likely to infect others in the community.

To improve the health of our population, greater emphasis must be placed on the promotion of health and the prevention of disease. The United States health-care system currently does not encourage preventive services to the extent that it should. Surgeons who perform amputations on people with diabetes are paid huge sums of money, while dietitians who provide nutritional and dietary counseling are paid very little. Insurance companies spend large amounts of money for gastric bypass and other types of bariatric surgery (and enable overweight people to become obese so that they qualify for such types of surgery), instead of diverting that money to preventative care and nutrition education. With the focus in this country on quick fixes, such as prescription drugs, both doctors and consumers often overlook the vast amount of research showing that regular exercise, not smoking, and a healthful diet are the best ways to prevent illness and diseases; however, these simple steps do not generate large profits for the insurance industry.

Investing in the prevention of diseases before they begin reduces the cost of health care later on. A 2008 report by the Trust for America's Health concluded that spending just $10 per person each year on effective, community-based preventive health programs could save the United States more than $16 billion per year within just 5 years.

The average American family spends between $10,000 and $12,000 every year for health insurance and other health-care needs. If that family could instead invest this money in a typical mutual fund account, the family would have about $1 million in the account within 20 to 25 years.

Health care and health insurance *must* become a right, just as public education is, instead of a privilege only for the wealthy. The American ideal of life, liberty, and the pursuit of happiness can never be reached for working-class people, for the elderly, for many who already are ill, or for the poor until every person in this country has access to adequate health care.

Health-Care Discrimination

As mentioned earlier, many people who belong to racial, ethnic, tribal, or religious minority groups may also face health-care discrimination, in addition to barriers caused by language and cultural beliefs. Health-care providers are sometimes unfamiliar with the special health needs of patients from backgrounds that are unlike their own, and many patients are uncomfortable discussing health issues and undergoing examination by a doctor or other health professional who is not a member of their cultural or ethnic group.

A patient's cultural and ethnic identity, habits, and beliefs can give doctors important clues about the patient's dietary, behavioral, and genetic risk factors for disease. Many genetic disorders have higher rates of incidence among specific segments of the population. In addition, responses to medications may also vary based on genetics, and therefore new treatments for some diseases are now being targeted for specific groups of patients.

Some examples of diseases that are related to genetics include the following:

- Tay Sachs disease is a fatal neurological disease that is diagnosed in children and occurs most often among people whose ancestors were Jews from Eastern Europe.
- Sickle cell anemia is most common among people with African and Mediterranean heritages.

As a result of barriers that prevent adequate access to health care, ethnic and racial minority groups tend to have a worse health status than that of the general population. Members of minority groups may also unintentionally receive substandard care because medical research tends to focus on conditions that commonly occur within the general population, rather than on diseases that typically affect smaller, minority populations.

> *"Public health practice is heavily burdened by the problem of inadvertent discrimination. For example, outreach activities may 'assume' that all populations are reached equally by a single, dominant-language message on television; or analysis 'forgets' to include health problems uniquely relevant to certain groups, like breast cancer or sickle cell disease; or a problem 'ignores' the actual response capability of different population groups, as when lead poisoning warnings are given without concern for financial ability to ensure lead abatement. Indeed, inadvertent discrimination is so prevalent that all public health policies and programs should be considered discriminatory until proven otherwise, placing the burden on public health to affirm and ensure its respect for human rights." (World Health Organization)*

Types of Health Insurance

A **health insurance policy** is a contract between a private company (or the government) and a person, whereby the company agrees to pay for certain health-care costs in exchange for regular payments, called premiums, by the person to the company. In the United States, health care is administered by a variety of providers that practice in different settings.

Types of Managed Care

Preferred provider organizations (PPOs) enter into contracts with providers to offer health-care services at discounted prices to all people who are covered by the PPO's plan. Patients who are covered by PPOs can choose a provider who does not participate in the plan but must then pay the difference in cost between the chosen provider and the preferred provider. Exclusive provider organizations (EPOs) are similar to PPOs, except that participants in an EPO must use the EPOs' providers or pay for the entire cost of health-care services themselves.

Health maintenance organizations (HMOs) combine health-care insurance and the provision of medical services into a single package. Members of HMOs pay monthly fees in exchange for the health care services that they need. There are several models of HMOs. In staff-model HMOs, doctors who provide medical services to HMO members are employees of the HMO and do not treat patients who do not belong to the HMO. In group-model HMOs, a doctors' group practice enters into a contract with an HMO to provide medical care to the HMO's members, but the doctors in the group practice may also treat patients who are not members. In the network-model HMO, two or more doctors' group practices enter into contracts with an HMO to provide medical service for the HMO's members and may also treat other patients. Finally, in the independent-practice-association HMO model, individual doctors enter into a contract with an HMO to provide health care for members of the HMO at a fixed fee for each HMO member.

Governmental Health Insurance

Medicare is health insurance provided by the federal government for Americans who are 65 years of age and older. The program is administered by the Health Care Financing Administration (HCFA). Medicare uses a pricing system in which health-care providers are paid a predetermined amount of money based on the specific diagnosis of the patient.

Medicare has several parts. Part A covers hospital care for all those 65 years old or older. Part B covers doctor visits and costs those who sign up for it $78 per month. Almost all Americans age 65 or older are covered by Parts A and B. Medicare Part C allows people age 65 and older to enroll in an HMO for Medicare, which can provide them with prescription drugs. Medicare Part D requires senior citizens to compare health-care plans—up to 85 in one area—and choose one plan based on a number of different factors. Seniors often are completely confused by this requirement of Medicare Part D, hence the nickname "D" for *Disaster.*

Medicaid is government-sponsored health insurance for poor and low-income individuals and families. Eligibility for the program is determined by each state, and there are no age requirements. Families and individuals who cannot afford to allocate one-third of their income to health insurance have no other health-care option but Medicaid. The cost of Medicaid has risen between 9% to 12% every year for the past five years, while at the same time, state budgets have been cut.

State Children's Health Insurance Program (SCHIP)

SCHIP is a program that is administered by the United States Department of Health and Human Services. The program provides matching funds to states for health insurance for families with children. The program was designed to cover uninsured children who are members of families with incomes that are fairly low but still too high to qualify for Medicaid. During the Bush administration, two Congressional bills designed to expand funding for SCHIP failed when then-President Bush vetoed the bills. In February of 2009, President Obama signed legislation that expanded SCHIP to include an additional 4 million children and pregnant women, and, for the first time, includes legal immigrants without a waiting period.

Prescription Drug Marketing

Americans pay an estimated 70% more for prescription drugs than do Canadians and Western Europeans. Prescription drugs are powerful substances. When they are taken for the right conditions, they can improve health and save lives, but when they are taken by the wrong person or for the wrong condition, they can be fatal. Unfortunately, doctors in the United States often do not receive complete and accurate information about new drugs that will enable them to make appropriate decisions about prescriptions, because drug manufacturers that wage aggressive marketing campaigns are one of the major sources of information for doctors. With managed care and cuts in Medicare reimbursements, many hospitals, laboratories, and universities do not have the funds to support research on new drugs. However, pharmaceutical companies do have a lot money, and thus they are the ones that provide financing for drug research. Pharmaceutical companies finance approximately 70% of the drug trials that are performed in the United States. Many Americans know that the pharmaceutical industry has one of the highest profit margins among the Fortune 500 companies.

The influence of the pharmaceutical industry can be seen everywhere, from the sponsoring of continuing medical education to the latest treatment guidelines. Their well-crafted television ads often convince viewers that they have disorders or diseases, when in fact they do not. One example of this is an ad campaign for hormone replacement therapy. Premarin was approved by the Food and Drug Administration (FDA) for the treatment of symptoms of menopause. The drug was originally created to treat specific women for only a few years, but the pharmaceutical company Wyeth-Ayerst began to market the drug as Hormone Replacement Therapy (HRT) and convinced millions of women that menopause was a disease. Years later, studies were finally released that showed that women who had taken the drug had increased risks of heart disease, breast cancer, dementia, stroke, blood clots, and other conditions and diseases. Even after the studies were released, HRT continued to be advertised on television.

More than 20 million Americans, including more than a million teenagers and children, take antidepressants or ADHD medications, such as Ritalin, Adderall, Prozac, Paxil, Effexor or Zoloft.

Do Americans really believe that about one out of every seven children should be taking these drugs?

Harvard physician Joseph Glenmullen has led the charge to warn the public about the dangers of antidepressants: they are over-prescribed, under-regulated, and often misunderstood in the side effects and withdrawal effects that they can produce. Now, antidepressants come with FDA-mandated warning labels that state that these drugs may cause agitation, anxiety, hostility, and even violent or suicidal tendencies. In 2003, the British government issued warnings and virtually banned many antidepressants for use by children and adolescents under age 18. The warnings were issued against the drugs because of evidence in the pharmaceutical companies' own studies that some of the antidepressants were no more effective for children than were placebos but in fact could cause children to become agitated, sleepless, hostile, aggressive, and even suicidal. In contrast, despite requiring that warnings be issued with prescriptions for antidepressants, the FDA has not banned any of these drugs for any age groups.

Some pharmaceutical companies have actually tried to suppress the warnings, specifically, the warning that antidepressants can increase suicidal thoughts and tendencies in children.

Instead of being prescribed safe and equally or more effective alternative drugs, millions of people in the United States are given prescriptions for drugs whose risks are dangerously understated. The crux of this problem is that the entirety of the information that the drug companies and the FDA have is not disclosed to consumers. This situation is unacceptable for the future of Americans' health.

How Other Countries Provide Health Care

National health insurance implies a system in which the federal government ensures that health care services are available for all people and that these services are paid for by tax dollars. Most developed countries have such health-care systems.

Canadian Health Care System

The Canadian health-care system addresses the problem of universal access to health care first, and then addresses its cost. In other words, each Canadian province must make sure that all its residents have access to medical care. The costs of this care are covered by a combination of public funds from provincial, federal, and corporate taxes, and from private funds. Canadian doctors are independent providers. As a result, Canadians spend much less on health care than Americans do, and there is a greater focus on prevention and primary care and less focus on specialized care.

National Health Services in Britain

The National Health Service (NHS) was established in 1948 to provide free health care for the citizens of the United Kingdom. The NHS is recognized as one of the best health-care services in the world by the World Health Organization. The most important feature of the service for its founders was that it was free at the point of need. The NHS is funded through general taxes and is administered by the national Department of Health. The UK also has private health-care providers, and people can opt to pay for private health care either through health insurance or when they use the services of these providers. Doctors are offered monetary incentives to help patients to reduce their weight, blood pressure and cholesterol levels.

Cuba's Socialized Healthcare

In 1976, the revised Cuban constitution stated that "Everyone has a right to health protection and care." In the movie *Sicko,* American filmmaker Michael Moore claims that the Cuban health-care system is far superior to that of the United States. Cubans spend, on average, 1/25 less on health care as Americans do, and their health care is free for all. In *Sicko,* Michel Moore features a woman who formerly had a good job but was bankrupted by her medical bills and forced to live with her daughter. She paid $240 a month for cancer medication in the United States but gets the same pills in Cuba for 10 cents each. Michael Moore's production company also took along a number of Ground Zero responders who were ill to be treated in Cuba, because Cuban doctors had developed new techniques for treating lung cancer and other respiratory illness.

Members of a study seminar from the American Public Health Association have also visited Cuba, and they have seen both the problems and the strengths of the Cuban health-care system. Cuba currently has more than 2,000 health-care professionals who provide aid in 57 other countries. Cuba's uniquely resourceful health-care system has continued to function well for decades, despite the U.S. embargo. Their focus on preventive care has resulted in greatly improved health indicators. For example, the incidence of infectious diseases that are preventable by vaccines is lower in Cuba than in any other nation at Cuba's level of economic development, because for many years, the rates of immunization have remained at between 99% and 100% of the target populations. Cuba has also implemented computerized surveillance at all provincial levels and is extending it to include municipalities and rural health-care centers. This surveillance quickly identifies problems such as the spread of infectious diseases and changes in the distribution of chronic diseases. Such innovations may be instructive for countries, including the

United States that lack efficient data gathering and reporting systems for preventive services and efforts directed toward community-oriented primary care.

Cuba's difficulty in obtaining petroleum products motivated the import of more than a million bicycles, which have significantly reduced traffic congestion and pollution, in addition to improving the overall physical health of Cubans. Similarly, the scarcity of red meat in Cuba has led to relatively low rates of cholesterol and blood lipids. Despite the U.S embargo on Cuba, which limits medicine and other supplies, all Cubans still receive free essential health care services.

Proactive Patients

Each person is ultimately in charge of his or her own health care, and everyone wants the best medical care possible. A proactive patient is an informed patient, one who finds a good doctor and medical facilities, does independent research using reliable sources, and asks detailed, relevant questions of health-care experts. The relationship between a patient and his or her doctors should be a partnership in which communication in central.

A proactive patient has three main attributes:

- knowledge about one's own health problems,
- assertiveness, and
- the willingness to participate in informed decision-making about one's own health care.

Providers must be sensitive to patients' beliefs and cultural values as they collaborate about health decisions. Proactive patients take some responsibility for obtaining their own information about health care so that it is accessible to them, and they understand their own health histories. Proactive patients engage in self-advocacy by being their own advocates: they represent their own interests in the health-care decision-making process by asking key questions, searching for information, and ensuring that they receive proper care.

How to get the most from your health care by being a proactive patient:

- Know your rights as a patient.
- Find out about informed-consent procedures, living wills, the durable power of attorney, organ donation, and other legal issues *before* you become ill.
- Ask about alternative procedures and about your treatment plans.

> *"The right to health does not mean the right to be healthy, nor does it mean that poor governments must put in place expensive health services for which they have no resources. But it does require governments and public authorities to put in place policies and action plans which will lead to available and accessible healthcare for all in the shortest possible time. To ensure that this happens is the challenge facing both the human rights community and public health professionals."*
>
> ***—United Nations High Commissioner for Human Rights Mary Robinson***

References

Abramson, John, *Overdosed America: The Broken Promise of American Medicine* (New York, Harper Collins s, 2004).

ABC News/Kaiser Family Foundation/*USA Today, "Health Care in America 2006 Survey,* October 17, 2006.

Agency for Healthcare Research and Quality, "Out-of-Pocket Expenditures on Health Care and Insurance Premiums among the Non-Elderly Population 2003," March 2006.

Aoki, Naomi, "Journals pool clout to ensure integrity," *The Boston Globe*, September 10, 2001.

Blendon, R.J., et al, "Understanding the American public's priorities: A 2006 perspective," *Health Affairs Web Exclusive* W508, 17 October, 2006.

Borger, C., et al., "Health spending projections through 2015: Changes on the horizon," *Health Affairs Web Exclusive* W61, 22 February 2006.

Boston at Risk, *Six Principles for a New Health Care System: A Blue Print for Action,* Families USA, 2006.

California Health Care Foundation, *Health Care Costs, Oakland:* March 2, 2005. http://www.chcf.org/topics/healthinsurance/index.cfm?subtopic=CL498&CFNoCache=TRUE&order=alpha

Catlin, A, C., Cowan, S., Heffler, et al, "National Health Spending in 2005," *Health Affairs* 26(1) (2006): 142–153.

Chernew, M, "Rising Health Care Costs and the Decline in Insurance Coverage," *Economic Research Initiative on the Uninsured,* ERTU Working Paper 8, September, 2002.

Committee on the Consequences of Uninsurance, *Health Insurance is a Family Matter.* (Washington, D.C.: *The National Academies Press,* 2002).

Eagan, Andrea Boroff, *The Women's Health Movement and Its Lasting Impact", An Unfinished Revolution, Women and Health Care in America,* Emily Friedman (ed.), (New York: United Hospital Fund of New York, 1994).

FamiliesUSA, at www.Farniliesusa.org.

Glenmullen, Joseph, *The Antidepressant Solution*, (New York: Free Press, January 9, 2006).

Health Care for All, *1995–2000 Annual Report, at* www.hcfa.org.

Hewitt Associates, LLC. *Health Care Expectations: Future State and Direction 2005.* November 17, 2004.

Himmelstein, D., E., Warren, D., Thorne, & S. Woolhander, "Illness and Injury as Contributors to Bankruptcy," *Health Affairs Web Exclusive* W5-63, February 2, 2005.

Langill, Donna, et al, *Medicaid Managed Care: An Advocate's Guide for Protecting Children,* Washington: (National Association of Children's Advocates and National Health Law Program, 1996) 115.

Marone, James, *The Democratic Wish, Popular Participation and the Limits of American Government* (New York: Basic Books, 1990).

McClellan, R. A., Burt, A. D., & Fleming, K. A., "Long-term safety and effectiveness of iron- chelation therapy with deferiprone for thalassemia major," *New England Journal of Medicine,* vol. 339 no. 7 (1998): 417–423.

McKinsey and Company, "Will Health Benefit Costs Eclipse Profits?" *The McKinsey Quarterly Chart Focus Newsletter,* September, 2004.

Meredith, Judy., & Dunham, Cathy. *Real Clout* (Boston: The Access Project, 1999).

Pear, R., "U.S. health care spending reaches all-time high: *15%* of GDP," *The New York Times,* January 9 2004, 3.

Schultz, Stacey, "True, false, whatever," *U.S. News & World Report,* September 17, 2001.

Seto, Natalie, and Weiskopf, Bess K., *Community Benefits, Need for Action, an Opportunity for Healthcare Change. A Workbook for Grassroots Leaders and Community Organizations* (Boston: The Access Project, 1998).

S. R. Collins, K. Davis, M. M. Doty, J. L. Kriss, & A. L. Holmgren, "Gaps in health insurance: An all-American problem," (New York: The Commonwealth Fund, April 2006).

Starr, Paul, *The Social Transformation of American Medicine* (New York: Basic Books, 1982).

The Commonwealth Fund, *Wages, Health Benefits, and Workers' Health,* Issue Brief, October 2004.

The Henry J. Kaiser Family Foundation, *Employee Health Benefits:2006 Annual Survey,* September 26, 2006.

The Henry J. Kaiser Family Foundation, *The Uninsured: A Primer, Key Facts About Americans without Health Insurance 2004,* November 10, 2004 .

The Henry J. Kaiser Family Foundation, *Health Care Worries in Context with Other Worries 2004,* October 4, 2004.

Public Health

NAME ______________________________ DATE ______________________

Assignment #7

1. Based on the criteria described in this chapter on the right to health, debate the issue of whether or not health care should be a right or a privilege. Offer your solutions.

2. Based on the three main attributes of being a proactive patient, do you consider yourself proactive? Describe your experiences or a family member's experiences with the U.S. medical system.

Chapter

8

CURRENT ISSUES IN GLOBAL HEALTH

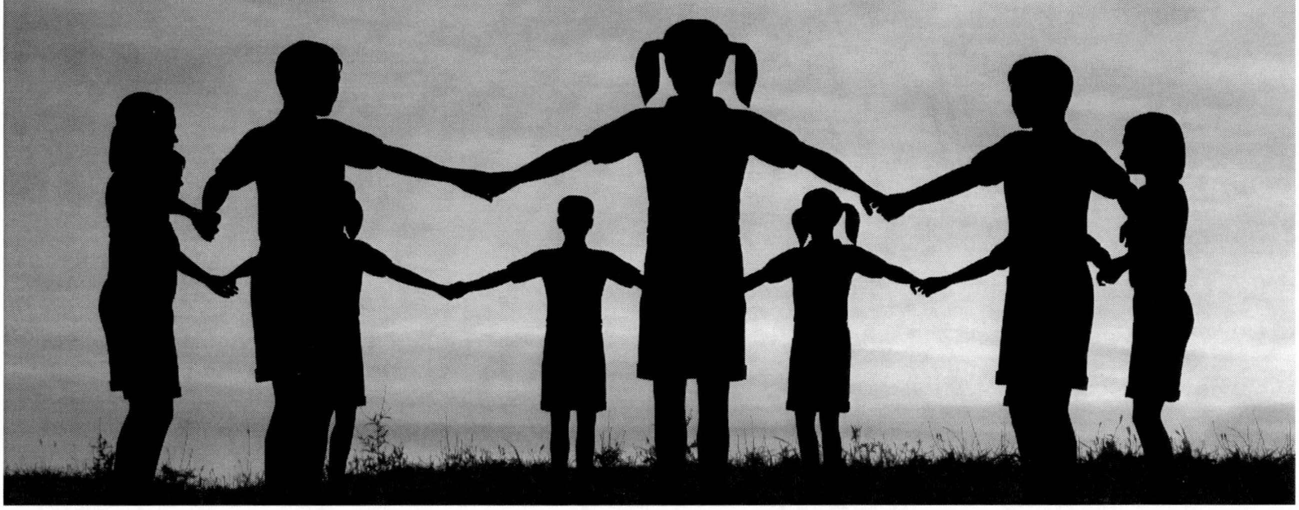

"The fact is that this generation—yours, my generation . . . we're the first generation that can look at poverty and disease, look across the ocean to Africa and say with a straight face, we can be the first to end this sort of stupid extreme poverty, where in the world of plenty, a child can die for lack of food in its belly. We have the cash, we have the drugs, and we have the science. Do we have the will to make poverty history?"

—*Bono*

Many people, mostly in tropical countries of the Third World, die every day from preventable, curable diseases, such as malaria, tuberculosis, and AIDS. The toll on the world's population that is taken by infectious diseases is enormous: almost 33 million people around the world live with HIV/AIDS, an estimated 14 million people live with tuberculosis, and approximately 250 million people live with malaria. These people are dying because the drugs needed to treat these illnesses either do not exist or are unavailable. Despite incredible advances in medicine and health since the 1950s, many challenges remain, which should have already been solved.

Declaration at the 2000 United Nations Millennium Summit

World leaders from both rich and poor countries committed to eight goals that, once they are achieved, will end extreme poverty worldwide by the year 2015. It is crucial that the wealthier countries hold up their end of the bargain, including more aid and more-effective aid, more sustainable debt relief, and fairer trade rules, before 2015. As of now, the richest countries collectively spend only half the amount (as a proportion of their national income) on international aid that they spent in the early 1960s, and only about 40% of that money actually reaches the countries for which it is intended.

Millennium Development Goals

1. Eradicate extreme poverty and hunger.
2. Achieve universal primary education.
3. Promote gender equality and empower women.
4. Reduce child mortality rates.
5. Improve maternal health.
6. Combat HIV/AIDS, malaria, and other diseases.
7. Ensure environmental sustainability.
8. Develop a global partnership for development.

If Current Trends Are Allowed To Continue,

- 45 million more children will die between now and 2015.
- 247 million more people in sub-Saharan Africa will be living on less than $1 a day in 2015.
- 97 million more children will not be in school in 2015.
- 53 million more people will lack proper sanitation facilities in 2015.

Goal: Eradicate extreme poverty and hunger

Did You Know?

- About one-third of deaths—about 18 million people each year, or 50,000 each day—are from poverty-related causes.
- Every year, more than 10 million children die of hunger and preventable diseases—equal to more than 30,000 people per day and one every 3 seconds.
- More than 1 billion people survive on less than $1 a day, with almost half of the world's population of 2.8 billion surviving on less than $2 a day.
- About 600 million children live in conditions of absolute poverty.
- The three richest people in the world control more wealth than all 600 million people who live in the world's poorest countries.
- The income per person in the poorest countries in Africa has fallen by a one-fourth in the past few decades.
- An estimated 800 million people go to bed hungry every day.

Factors for Global Poverty

- overcrowded cities and, poor sanitation,
- a lack of access to health care and medicine,
- poor food quality,
- urban air pollution,
- the drug trade and the sex trade, and
- a lack of education.

Top Ten Global Health Priorities

1. Ensure healthier mothers and children.
2. Stop the AIDS pandemic.
3. Promote good nutrition.
4. Decrease the rates of tuberculosis.
5. Control malaria.
6. Reduce the toll from cardiovascular disease.
7. Combat tobacco use.
8. Reduce fatal and disabling injuries.
9. Ensure equal access to quality health care.
10. Form strong, integrated, effective health-care systems.

Malaria, HIV/AIDS, and tuberculosis are among the diseases that disproportionately affect the world's poorest populations, which places a huge burden on the economies of developing countries.

Malaria

Malaria is a life-threatening parasitic disease that is transmitted by mosquitoes. The parasite infects a a person from the bite of a female Anopheles mosquito, which requires blood to nurture her eggs. The infected person then transmits the disease to other people, who in turn transmit it to others. Malaria can kill people by destroying their red blood cells, causing anemia, and by clogging the capillaries that carry blood to the brain (cerebral malaria) or to other vital organs.

In Africa, malaria is both a disease of poverty and a cause of poverty. An African child dies every 30 seconds from malaria. Many children who do survive a case of severe malaria may suffer from learning impairments or brain damage. When the necessary drugs are not available or the parasites are resistant to the drugs, a malarial infection can progress rapidly to become life-threatening. Displaced people, such as refugees, who live in makeshift housing, are especially vulnerable to malaria, because they are more likely to be bitten by mosquitoes, are often already ill with other infections, and lack access to adequate health care.

The human costs of malaria include the following:

- a loss of productivity,
- lost income associated with illness and death,
- human pain and suffering caused by the disease,
- negative consequences for children's schooling and social development both because of absenteeism and permanent neurological and other damage associated with severe cases of the disease.

Malaria is largely preventable and 100% treatable. Many poor people who do not have access to such basic preventable measures as bed nets treated with insecticide will die from the disease. Such a bed net costs only $5. One day's worth of spending on the military budget of the United States would provide all sleeping sites in Africa with five years of bed-net coverage, which would eradicate a disease that kills millions every year.

Priority Actions

- Provide universal access to insecticide-treated bed nets.
- Spray indoor surfaces with long-lasting insecticides.
- Provide funding for more effective drugs.

Tuberculosis

Tuberculosis (TB) is a contagious respiratory disease that is spread through the air. When people become infected with TB, it is usually from a cough, sneeze, talk or spit, released into the air by TB bacilli. A person need only inhale a small number of these bacilli to become infected. Symptoms of TB include fever, weight loss, night sweats, and the coughing up of blood. However, people who are infected with TB bacilli do not necessarily experience symptoms of the disease right away. The body's immune system can hide the TB bacilli, which are protected by a thick waxy coat, and they can lie dormant for years. When a person's immune system becomes weakened, the chances of the person becoming ill from the TB bacilli increase.

As especially dangerous form of TB is multidrug-resistant TB (MDR-TB), which is the disease caused by TB bacilli that is resistant to anti-TB drugs. MDR-TB is caused by inconsistent or partial treatment for the disease, as, for example, when patients do not take all their prescribed medicines regularly and for the necessary period because they feel better; because doctors or other health workers administer the wrong treatment regimens; or because the drug supply is unreliable. The fatality rate for MDR-TB is six times higher than the rate for non-MDR-TB.

Approximately one-third of the world's population is currently infected with TB bacilli. Many people likely would be shocked and saddened to learn that one of leading causes of death throughout the world is a disease for which treatment has been available since the mid-twentieth century with rates of recovery of about 95%.

Priority Actions

- Treat active TB cases quickly.
- Manage multidrug resistant TB with new drugs and drug combinations.
- Provide free access for testing and treatment.
- Develop a low-cost vaccine against pulmonary TB.

Global AIDS

Did You Know?

- In Africa, 6,500 people die of AIDS every day, and another 9,500 contract the HIV virus,1,400 of which are newborns who are infected during childbirth or by their mothers' milk.
- So far, more than 11 million African children have lost at least one parent to HIV/AIDS; that number is expected to reach 20 million by the year 2010.
- About 5 people die every minute from AIDS.
- Almost 3 million children are living with AIDS, and more than 4 million have died of AIDS since the epidemic began.
- About 1 in every 100 people worldwide is HIV positive, and one-third of these are between the ages of 15 and 24.

HIV (human immunodeficiency virus) is the virus that causes AIDS. This virus can be transmitted from one person to another when infected blood, semen, or vaginal secretions come in contact with an uninfected person's broken skin or mucous membranes. Pregnant women who are infected with HIV can pass it on to their babies during pregnancy or delivery, and mothers of newborns can transmit the virus to their babies through breast-feeding.

The most common ways in which HIV spreads are through sexual contact, the sharing of needles for illicit drug use, and transmission from infected mothers to babies. The transmission of HIV through sexual contact can occur from men to men, men to women, women to men, and women to women through vaginal, anal, and oral sex. The best way to prevent sexual transmission of HIV is abstinence from sexual contact until both partners in a monogamous relationship are certain that they are not infected with HIV. Because an HIV antibody test can take up to

6 months to indicate a positive result, both partners should test negative 6 months after their last potential exposure to HIV before having sexual relations. Aside from abstinence, the use of latex condoms is the next-best method of preventing the spread of HIV through sexual contact.

Symptoms of HIV first became noticed in 1981 among homosexual men in Los Angeles and New York. These men had an unusual type of pneumonia and rare skin tumors called Kaposi's sarcoma. They also had dangerously low levels of T cells in their blood. T cells are an important part of the immune system and help the body fight infections. In 1985, a blood test became available to measure antibodies to HIV that are the body's immune response to the HIV virus. Currently, tests are available to detect these same antibodies in saliva and urine; some can provide results within 20 minutes of testing.

HIV is a virus that infects the body's cells and makes new copies of itself within those cells. The virus can also damage human cells, which is one of the ways in which it can cause a person to become ill. As time goes on, a person who is infected with HIV is likely to become ill more and more often. At some point, usually several years after they became infected, they are afflicted with one of a variety of severe illnesses, which ultimately will kill them. A person does not die of AIDS, but rather from complications of common diseases, such as a cold, the flu, or pneumonia, because at that stage of HIV infection, the body's immune system has very little defense against any kind of infection.

Approximately 42 million people around the world are now living with HIV and AIDS, which respect no borders, no economic class, no gender, and no age. The fact that health-care services in poor countries lack doctors and nurses, combined with the high price of drugs, means that the vast majority of poor people have no access to treatment. More than 20 million people have died of complications from AIDS since the disease was first identified in 1981, and about 3 million people current die from such complications every year.

However, many countries, including Brazil, Uganda, and Thailand, have been successful in reducing rates of HIV infection. Politicians are increasingly making a commitment to fight the spread of the disease in their countries, and medicines to treat it are becoming increasingly available in poor countries. Still, the incidence of AIDS remains incredibly high in Africa. The disease is now spreading most quickly in Eastern Europe and Asia, which includes about 60% of the world's population.

Russia

Russia is experiencing one of the fastest-growing rates of infection in the world, with an estimated 1 million Russians being HIV positive. The World Bank projects that by the year 2020, the number of HIV cases in Russia could range anywhere between 5.4 million to 14.5 million.

More than 80% of Russians infected with HIV are under the age of 30, most often as a result of the sharing of infected needles for illicit drug use. Because the unauthorized possession of needles and syringes is illegal in Russia, many drug users share needles and then engage in unprotected sex, which spreads the HIV virus into the general population.

In addition, there are many sex workers in Russia and other parts of Eastern Europe, many of whom work in exchange for drugs or to get money to buy drugs. Sex workers regularly engage in sexual relations with multiple partners, and they may or may not use protection. In addition, prisons in the region are often overcrowded and unsanitary, with a large number of prisoners being illicit drug users. Of these prisoners, a majority of them continue to use drugs and share needles while in prison, and also to engage in unprotected sex.

China

The Chinese government has stated that an estimated 650,000 people in China are living with HIV, including about 75,000 AIDS patients. UNAIDS and other organizations have predicted that by 2010, China could experience a generalized epidemic, with between 10 and 20 million people who are HIV positive.

> *"Exact figures are difficult to arrive at because governments at local levels are very reticent to report on actual cases, a situation compounded by individuals who are reluctant to come forward because of discrimination."*
>
> *—Qi Xiaoqiu, Director of China's Department of Disease Control*

Most HIV infections that have occurred in China have been attributed to drug use with infected needles, commercial blood or plasma donations, or sexual contact. At one time, poor rural farmers in several Chinese provinces sold their blood and plasma to commercial blood-processing companies to supplement their incomes. These companies operated illegally for the most part and sold blood products both internationally and domestically.

The challenge that China now faces is to educate people about the proper use of condoms and also to provide enough condoms of good quality. Fear and discrimination cause people to hide the fact that they are infected, information is scarce, and counseling and care are often not available. All of these factors create a vicious cycle that fuels the HIV/AIDS epidemic.

In 2003, the Chinese government launched China CARES (China Comprehensive AIDS Response), a community-based, HIV treatment, care, and prevention program. The goals of the program include the following:

- to provide free anti-HIV medication to AIDS patients who are rural residents or who live in urban areas and have financial difficulties;
- to provide free voluntary counseling and testing; and
- to provide free medication to HIV-infected pregnant women so as to prevent mother-to-child transmission, as well as HIV testing for newborns.

Thailand

In Thailand, a "100% condom program" has been initiated. The goal of this program is to control HIV, and since its inception, it has cut visits to sex workers in half. The program entails the enforcement of consistent condom use in all commercial sex establishments. Condoms are distributed without charge to all brothels and massage parlors, and all sex workers and their clients are required to use them. Brothels that fail to comply with these requirements are shut down.

India

After Africa, India has the second-highest number of people who are infected with HIV, with about 5.1 million known cases. Knowledge and education about HIV is still not widespread in India, and an underlying problem of bisexual men infecting women exists. In addition, some truck drivers patronize HIV-infected prostitutes and then infect their wives. Educating India's population about HIV/AIDS and how it can be prevented is a particularly difficult task, because several major languages and hundreds of different dialects are spoken by people who live in the country.

Some Indians who have HIV also face societal discrimination and punishment. Many of them have been subject to violent attacks; have been shunned by their families, spouses, and communities; have been refused medical treatment; and even reportedly have been denied the last rites of their religion before they die. Some AIDS outreach workers and peer-educators have reported harassment, and teachers sometimes must deal with the negative reactions of the parents of school children whom they teach about HIV/AIDS.

Under the second stage of Indian's National AIDS Control Program, which ended in March of 2006, the government granted funding to AIDS-prevention groups for, among other things, educational youth campaigns, blood safety checks, and HIV testing. A variety of public platforms was used to raise awareness of the epidemic, including concerts, radio dramas, a day devoted to voluntary blood donation, and TV spots featuring a popular Indian film star. The schools also conveyed educational messages about HIV to young people. Teachers and peer-educators had been trained to teach about the subject, and students were educated through active learning sessions, including debates and role-playing. The Indian government announced that this campaign would place a strong emphasis on the use of condoms. It has already supported the installation of more than 11,000 condom vending machines in colleges, roadside restaurants, gas stations, and hospitals.

Latin America

At the end of 2005, an estimated 1.6 million people were living with HIV in Latin America. Of these, more than half resided in the region's four largest countries: Brazil, Mexico, Columbia, and Argentina, with Brazil having the highest number—600,000 people. In nearly every Latin American country, the highest levels of HIV infection are found among men who have sex with other men. However this remains a largely hidden problem, because homophobia and a culture of machismo are common throughout the region, and sex between men is highly stigmatized.

Sex workers and drug users also play major roles in the spread of HIV in several Latin American countries. In addition, migration occurs on a large scale throughout Latin America, and several factors may place migrants in this region at a high risk of HIV infection, including poverty, a lack of adequate health-care services, a high level of risk-taking, rape and other types of violence, and contact with sex workers in different areas of the region.

For decades, a violent civil conflict between left-wing guerrilla groups and right-wing paramilitaries has raged in Colombia. An economic downturn, widespread violence including torture and murder, and drug trafficking are just parts of the large-scale suffering that the Columbian people have endured as a result of the fighting. Gay men, the group most affected by Colombia's HIV/AIDS epidemic, have faced violence and oppression from both sides of the conflict.

Some of the most effective HIV/AIDS prevention efforts have occurred in Brazil, where societal groups and other nongovernmental organizations have helped to fight the stigma of AIDS and to raise awareness about the disease. In addition, the government itself has actively promoted the use of condoms in media campaigns and advertisements. It has also distribued large numbers of free condoms—25 million in 2006 alone. HIV prevention efforts in Brazil have targeted high-risk groups, such as sex workers and men who have sex with men. In addition, needle-exchange stations have been established in a number of areas, which has helped to reduce the incidences of HIV infection among intravenous drug users.

The Caribbean

The Caribbean country with the highest rate of infection is Haiti, with 5.6% of the population afflicted with the virus. Cuba has the lowest rate of HIV, with only 0.1% of the population infected.

In the Caribbean, HIV is spread mostly through heterosexual sex, often involving prostitution. However, in addition to sex workers, men who have sex with men are also a high-risk group, although this is largely a hidden population. Both groups are highly stigmatized and not generally recognized as part of mainstream society.

> *"Gays and lesbians in Jamaica exist with the possibility that you might be chased, you might be run down, you might be killed because of your sexual orientation, and when a day ends when that does not happen, we give thanks."*
>
> *—Gareth Williams, the Jamaica Forum for Lesbians, All-Sexuals and Gays (JFLAG)*

Intravenous drug use is a major cause of HIV transmission in Bermuda and Puerto Rico. In Puerto Rico, many experts believe that there is an urgent need for more needle-exchange stations and methadone treatment clinics, both of which have proven to be effective in many other countries in reducing the rate of HIV transmission among intravenous drug users.

Cuba once took the controversial approach of mandatory testing for HIV for certain groups within the population, including pregnant women, hospital patients, and prison inmates. When testing revealed that people were HIV positive, they were placed in sanatoriums, where they were provided with care and support while their sexual partners were traced. These methods have certainly been successful, as infection rates in Cuba have remained exceptionally low. Cuba's preventive mother-to-child-transmission program is one of the most effective in the world; all pregnant women are tested for HIV, and those who test positive are immediately treated with antiretroviral medication to reduce the risk of transmission to their babies.

Cuba is now the only country in the Caribbean with universal access to HIV medication. However, for many years, Cubans did not have access to such medication because of the U.S. embargo, which prevents trade between the Cuban government and U.S. pharmaceutical companies and their foreign-based subsidiaries. To overcome this problem, Cuban scientists developed generic versions of the medications, which are now manufactured in Cuba. There is now an ample supply of these generic medications for all Cubans who need them. In fact, the Cuban government has offered to supply antiretroviral medicines to other Caribbean nations, as well as to send doctors and nurses to help in their fight against HIV/AIDS.

Africa

In sub-Saharan Africa, there are an estimated 25 million people infected with HIV. In some African countries, life expectancies have fallen below 40 years of age. Most AIDS-related deaths occur among young adults, which have devastating effects on families, communities, and economies.

Factors that influence the rate at which HIV is transmitted in Africa include the following:

- poverty;
- social instability;
- gender inequality;
- sexual violence;
- other sexually transmitted infections, which facilitate HIV transmission;
- high rates of mobility;
- rapid urbanization and modernization; and
- ineffective leadership.

Some of the cultural and traditional practices of certain groups in Africa, for example, drying the vagina before sexual intercourse, increase the likelihood of abrasions, which in turn increases the risk of the HIV virus being transmitted. Another high-risk cultural behavior is the belief among some groups that a male who has sex with a virgin will rid his body of HIV/AIDS.

A lack of male circumcision is another contributor to the spread of HIV in Africa. Very strong evidence now exists that circumcised men are about half as likely as uncircumcised men to acquire HIV through heterosexual sex. This is an example of cultural practices that can either reduce or increase the spread of HIV.

Another cultural belief that exists in some parts of Africa is AIDS denialism (a theory that denies the existence of AIDS). President Thabo Ivibeki of South Africa is one such believer, and his administration is not active in expanding access to antiretroviral drugs. Instead, it promotes nutritional alternatives such as lemons, garlic, and olive oil to treat HIV infections. Thousands of South Africans are dying after changing their diets rather than taking antiretroviral medication.

Medical advances have enabled HIV-infected people who live in wealthy countries to obtain treatment and to live longer lives; however, these treatments are still unavailable to an estimated 70% of Africans who are infected with HIV. Drug manufacturing companies in the United States and Europe control the supply of AIDS medications, and they keep the prices of these medications high so that they can make large profits.

HIV/AIDS in the United States

In the United States, HIV/AIDS began in the early 1980s as an epidemic primarily viewed as affecting gay, white men. The epidemic has since changed in that it disproportionately affects African Americans. According to the Centers for Disease Control and Prevention (CDC), African Americans currently account for more than half of all HIV/AIDS cases in the United states, and HIV/AIDS is now the leading cause of death among African American women between the ages of 25 and 34. African American women in the United States are diagnosed with HIV/AIDS at a rate 23 times that for white women, while African American men are diagnosed at a rate 7 times higher than that for white men.

Women are at a disproportionately higher risk for contracting HIV for the following reasons:

- poverty;
- sexual abuse;
- married men secretly also having sex with other men;

- a lack of female-controlled HIV prevention methods;
- disparities in access to health care;
- imbalances of power; and
- threats of sexual violence (rape, incest, abuse), which deters women from trying to persuade men to practice safer sex or to resist unprotected sex.

Health officials who have been tracking the disproportionate rates of AIDS-related deaths among minorities over the past several years suggest that those rates are a result of such factors as a failure to identify those who are infected and provide them with treatment, a failure to persuade those who are being treated to continue with the treatment, and the strong stigma that AIDS has in many minority communities.

Children

More than half of all new HIV infections in the United States are now occurring in young people under the age of 25. Every minute of every day, a child under the age of 15 becomes infected with HIV. In most of these cases, the virus is transmitted by an HIV-infected mother to her fetus, during delivery, or through breastfeeding after birth. An estimated 90% of the more than 5 million children in the United States who are HIV-infected were born in Africa. The other most common causes of HIV infection in children include contaminated blood products or syringes and sexual abuse.

Prevention of maternal and childhood HIV:

- HIV prevention education and family planning for all women of childbearing age;
- counseling, testing, and access to antiretroviral treatment for all those infected;
- education on how to avoid unintended pregnancy;
- steps to reduce the risk of transmission during and after pregnancy;
- the direct confrontation of child sexual abuse;
- education and access to confidential, low-cost, and youth-friendly contraceptive services for sexually active youths to reduce teenage pregnancies and to help them protect themselves from sexually transmitted diseases and HIV infection.

Abstinence-Only Education

A national study completed in 2007 concluded that abstinence-only sex education does not prevent teenagers from having sex, nor does it have any affect on the likelihood that when they do have sex, they will use a condom. In contrast, responsible sex-education programs have been shown to have such positive results as teenagers delaying having sex, reducing the frequency of sexual encounters, and increasing contraceptive use.

The United States has unacceptably high rates of teenage pregnancies, sexually transmitted diseases (STDs), and HIV/AIDS infections. To address this problem, we must support age-appropriate and medically accurate health-education programs that promote abstinence *and* provide adolescents with the information that they need to protect themselves if they do choose to be sexually active. Research indicates that honest, medically accurate sex education works, while abstinence-only programs do not. Many abstinence-only programs include false and misleading information, which teenagers often pick up on.

Harm Reduction

Harm-reduction programs allow intravenous drug users to exchange dirty needles for sanitary needles. The thinking behind harm reduction programs is that if a clean supply of needles is available to intravenous drug users, they will be less likely to share needles with other users, thereby reducing the risk of infecting themselves and others with HIV.

HIV Medication

HIV is a type of virus called a retrovirus, and drugs that disrupt the action of HIV are called antiretrovirals. These have proven to be very effective in treating people with AIDS, but they cannot cure AIDS. HAART is a form of treatment that includes antiretrovirals drugs and significantly delays the progression from HIV to AIDS. HAART has been available in wealthy countries since 1996, but less-wealthy and poor countries, very few people who are HIV-positive can afford this treatment.

Access to treatment is one of the major concerns of people who are infected with HIV/AIDS, most of whom cannot afford the necessary health care and antiretrovirals. Access to drugs, to some degree, also depends upon people being aware of their HIV status, knowledgeable about treatment, and empowered to seek such treatment.

The Role of Big Pharmaceutical Companies

To some extent, HIV/AIDS is a disease of poverty. When poverty contributes to the spread of a disease or causes a disease in a community, large pharmaceutical companies benefit by holding power and influence, especially in poorer countries. One of the major reasons for unnecessary deaths worldwide is that people simply cannot afford life-saving medication that exists. Sadly, millions of people die from preventable or curable diseases every week.

Multinational pharmaceutical companies often ignore certain diseases in under-developed countries because there is no profit to be made there. Instead, these companies concentrate on producing more drugs that lead to high profits, such as new medications for headaches and erectile dysfunction.

A documentary entitled *Dying for Drugs* reveals how one of the world's largest pharmaceutical companies experimented on children in Africa without their parents' knowledge or consent. The film also showed how a drug company attempted to silence a prominent expert in Canada who had doubts about the efficacy or safety of a particular drug that the company manufactured. In South Korea, the documentary followed the attempts of desperately ill patients to convince a leading pharmaceutical company to provide them with life-saving drugs at a price that they could afford. Finally, the film showed a 12-year old Honduran child dying from AIDS and people trying to help him by smuggling the drugs that he needed across the Guatemalan border, breaking the law in the process, simply to obtain the drugs at affordable prices. The child died as the documentary crew was filming the desperate smuggling.

In India, patent laws allow the production of cheap generic drugs. The Chemical, Industrial & Pharmaceutical Laboratories (CIPLA) is a large Indian pharmaceutical company best-known outside of India for its manufacture and distribution of a low-cost antiretroviral for HIV-positive people in developing countries, even though the company took a loss in profit. Company representatives said that CIPLA made profits from other drugs, and that this undertaking was about more than a matter of profit and loss. However, the Indian government has been pressured about its patent laws by wealthy countries for a some time. When CIPLA offered to provide a cocktail of antiretroviral drugs for AIDS at the price of $350 a year, compared to the $10,000 charged by multinational pharmaceutical companies, this sent shockwaves to both large pharmaceutical companies and to poor countries. Poor countries realized that there actually was a more affordable way to deal with the HIV/AIDS health crisis, which afflicted them the most, while the large multinational drug companies saw their monopoly prices not only exposed, but also threatened.

As a result of the bad publicity generated by this incident, many large pharmaceutical companies began to offer AIDS antiretrovirals and other drugs at cheaper prices and even donated large amounts of money to global HIV/AIDS initiatives. Former President Clinton's HIV/AIDS Initiative (CHAI) has been working to lower the prices that people in developing countries have to pay for AIDS antiretrovirals. CHAI has become a major force in helping poor countries to negotiate prices with pharmaceutical companies and to obtain faster AIDS tests.

Priority actions to reduce the spread of HIV/AIDS include the following:

- Promote 100% condom use and education, especially among populations at high risk.
- Treat other sexually transmitted diseases that increase the risk of HIV infection.
- Provide antiretroviral medications, especially for pregnant women.
- Offer harm-reduction programs (e.g., needle exchanges) for intravenous drug users.
- Offer voluntary counseling and testing for HIV.
- Combat the stigma and discrimination surrounding HIV and AIDS.

Maternal and Child Health

Maternal and child health is one of the major subfields of public health. Child health professionals pay special attention to children in their first 5 years of life, who are most vulnerable to illnesses and death.

It is a disgrace that so many children die of diseases that are easily preventable. The silent killers are poverty and hunger, which are easily preventable.

More than 25,000 children die every day around the world, which is equivalent to

- 1 child dying every 3.5 seconds,
- 17–18 children dying every minute,
- a 2004 Asian Tsunami occurring almost every 1.5 weeks,

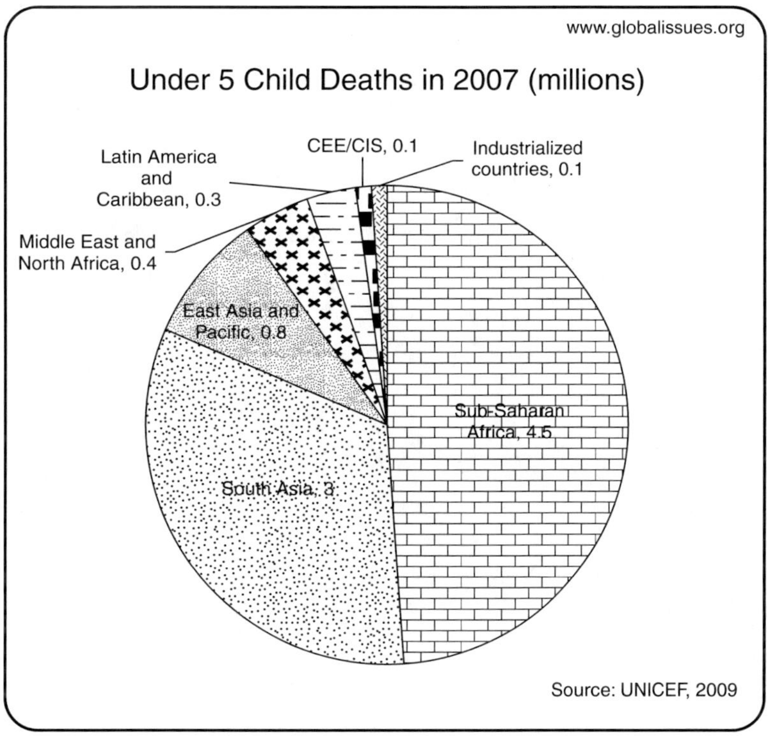

Goal: Reduce Child Mortality

Leading Causes of Death of Children Globally:

- malnutrition,
- pneumonia,
- diarrhea,
- measles, and
- malaria.

Factors for Deaths of Children Globally:

- **Poverty:** is the root cause of high rates of child mortality and morbidity. A lack of sanitation pollutes the water that children drink, and poor nutrition makes them vulnerable to illnesses and diarrhea, which, if untreated, can cause dehydration and further reduce a child's body weight and resistance to disease.
- **Armed conflicts:** As wars proliferate, hundreds of thousands of children are caught up in conflicts by being forced to become soldiers; being refugees; and suffering sexual violence, abuse, and exploitation. Even when children caught in conflicts are not killed or injured, they can be orphaned, abducted, raped, and left with emotional scars and trauma from direct exposure to violence or from dislocation and the loss of family members. Even when these conflicts end, there is still the danger of abandoned explosives and weapons, and landmines, which kill and maim thousands of children every year.
- **HIV/AIDS:** is the leading cause of death in the world for people aged 15 to 49. Every day, approximately 1,800 children, most of them newborns, become infected with HIV. Without HIV medication, about 45% of HIV-infected children die before they reach the age of 2. Often, the consumption of food in an AIDS-affected household declines, especially when the person suffering from AIDS is an adult who had previously helped to support the family. This leaves children at a higher risk for malnutrition and under-nutrition. Many children whose families are affected by HIV/AIDS, especially girls, are forced to drop out of school so that they can work or care for their families.
- **Trafficking and child labor:** An estimated 1.2 million children throughout the world are bought and sold every year, and about 2 million children, the majority of them girls, are exploited in the commercial sex industry. Some children are bought and forced to work in sweatshops or as farm workers harvesting coffee. Currently, approximately 180 million children are engaged in some form of child labor.

The trafficking of children often involves the exploitation of their parents' extreme poverty.

Parents may sell children to traffickers to pay off debts or to supplement their income; sometimes they are deceived about the prospects of education, training, and a better life than they can provide for their children. In West Africa, children who are sold have often lost one or both parents to AIDS.

- **Malnutrition and Under-Nutrition:** The WHO cites under-nutrition as the largest single contributor to the premature deaths of children. Infants who weigh less than 5.5 pounds at birth are at greater risk for diseases and death than are infants with a normal birth weight, which is about 8 pounds. Under-nutrition is an underlying cause of an estimated 53% of all deaths of children younger than age 5.

The first step in preventing the deaths of children is to make sure that every child is well nourished and has safe and adequate food and water.

- **Pneumonia:** in children under 5 years of age is the leading cause of childhood mortality in the world. More than 2 million children die from pneumonia every year, accounting for almost 1 out of 5 deaths of children under age 5 worldwide. Pneumonia is usually caused by an air-borne bacterial pathogen.

  Symptoms include: fever, cough, and rapid or difficult breathing

Early diagnosis and treatment of pneumonia with simple antibiotics can prevent a large number of deaths. The antibiotics needed to treat 20 children with pneumonia cost only $5.

The three main ways to prevent pneumonia from developing are the following:

- adequate nutrition, including breastfeeding infants,
- raising immunization rates, and
- reducing indoor air pollution.

Diarrhea: Millions of people do not have access to safe water and adequate sanitation, which increases their risk of contracting food- and water-borne diarrheal infections. Children are more vulnerable than adults are to the effects of diarrhea, because their immune systems are less able to respond to infections that cause diarrhea. Severe diarrhea in children may quickly lead to death.

Nearly all deaths from diarrhea can be prevented through the use of an inexpensive solution of glucose and sodium, which rehydrates the body.

To prevent exposure to the pathogens responsible for diarrhea, developing countries need to focus on the following:

- sanitation,
- hygiene, especially hand washing,
- access to clean water,
- access to safe food, and
- improved nutritional status.

Measles: is caused by a virus and is easily spread from person to person by contact with nasal or throat secretions through sneezing or coughing of infected persons. Until recently, measles killed nearly 900,000 children throughout the world every year. Following a joint WHO and UNICEF plan to expand the provision of measles vaccines, deaths from measles have declined.

Symptoms include: a high fever, coughing, a runny nose, and a generalized rash

Complications that can develop: pneumonia, diarrhea, malnutrition, and death

Prevention includes: vaccination, which is unavailable in many underdeveloped countries

Malaria: Four parasites cause malaria, and all are transmitted through the bite of an *Anopheles* mosquito. The majority of deaths from malaria occur among young children.

Symptoms include: fever, headache, and vomiting.

Prevention includes: the use of insecticide-treated bed nets and indoor spraying with insecticides to prevent mosquito bites

(Yet only 1 out of 25 children in sub-Saharan Africa sleeps under an insecticide-treated bed net.)

Solutions to Decreasing Deaths Globally of Children:

- Just 4 cents can protect and boost one child's immune system with vitamin A capsules.
- Just 6 cents can buy one packet of oral rehydration salts for one child for the treatment of severe dehydration and diarrhea, a leading cause of death among young children.
- Just $1 can buy 40 liters of safe drinking water, which is enough for one child to survive for 40 days, or for forty children to have safe drinking water for one day.
- Just $5 can provide a box of 100 disposable syringes for use during immunization campaigns, and $17 can immunize one child for life against six deadly diseases.
- Just $100 can provide ten families with insecticide-treated bed nets to protect them from malaria-carrying mosquitoes.

Major Causes of Child Deaths and the Cost to Treat or Prevent Illness

Disease	Percentage of deaths under five	Number of deaths annually	Cost to treat/prevent illness for one child	
Pneumonia	19 percent	2 million	Antibiotic treatment	$ 0.30
Diarrhea	17 percent	1.8 million	Oral rehydration packet	$ 0.20
Malaria	8 percent	850,000	Insecticide treated bed net	$ 5.00
Measles	4 percent	400,000	Measles vaccine	$ 1.10
HIV/AIDS	3 percent	350,000	Anti-retroviral drug	$ 5.00
Source: Global Health Council www.globalhealth.org				

Major Causes of Death for Women in the United States

1. Heart disease
2. Cancer
3. Stroke
4. Chronic lower-respiratory diseases
5. Alzheimer's disease
6. Unintentional injuries
7. Diabetes
8. Influenza and pneumonia
9. Kidney disease
10. Septicemia

In the United States, the biggest threats to women's health are largely preventable.

1. ***To prevent heart disease:***
   - Don't smoke. Avoid exposure to secondhand smoke.
   - Eat a healthful diet that is rich in vegetables, fruits, whole grains, fiber, and fish. Reduce your intake of foods high in saturated fats and sodium.
   - If you have high cholesterol or high blood pressure, carefully follow your doctor's treatment recommendations.
   - Include physical activity in your daily routine.
   - Maintain a healthful weight.
   - If you drink alcohol, do so only in moderation. Too much alcohol can raise blood pressure.
   - If you have diabetes, keep your blood sugar under control.
   - Manage stress.
2. ***To reduce the risk of cancer:***
   - Don't smoke. Avoid exposure to secondhand smoke.
   - Include physical activity in your daily routine.
   - Maintain a healthful weight.
   - Eat a healthful diet that is rich in fruits and vegetables, and avoid high-fat foods.
   - Limit your exposure to the sun. When you are outdoors, use sunscreen.
   - If you drink alcohol, do so only in moderation.
   - Consult your doctor for regular cancer screenings.
   - Reduce exposure to cancer-causing substances (carcinogens), such as radon, asbestos, radiation, and air pollution.
3. ***To reduce your risk of stroke:***
   - Don't smoke.
   - Limit the amount of saturated fats and cholesterol in your diet. Avoid trans fat entirely.
   - Maintain a healthful weight.
   - Include physical activity in your daily routine.
   - If you have diabetes, keep your blood sugar under control.
   - If you drink alcohol, do so only in moderation.

Did You Know?

- Of the 1.3 billion people living in poverty around the world, about 70% are women.
- Women do about 66% of the work throughout the world in exchange for less than 5% of its income.
- In the least-developed countries, nearly twice as many women as men over age 15 are illiterate.
- Two-thirds of children who do not have access to primary education are girls, and 75% of the world's 876 million illiterate adults are women.
- More than half a million women die during pregnancy and childbirth every year, which equals one death every minute. Of these deaths, 99% occur in developing countries. In parts of Africa, the maternal mortality rate is about1 out of 16 women.
- Only 28 of 100 women who are giving birth are attended by trained health personnel in the least-developed countries.

Causes of Death for Women Globally in Low Income Countries

1. **HIV/AIDS**
2. **Maternal conditions**
3. **Unintentional injuries**

Levels of maternal mortality reflect the disparities between the rich and the poor. Inadequate access to prenatal care, poverty, and gender inequality are the main causes of maternal mortality.

Factors for maternal mortality include the following:

- inadequate access to reproductive health services;
- unsafe abortions (43 million women per year have abortions; of these, half are unsafe);
- inadequate prenatal care;
- forced sex and inability to negotiate condom use; and
- gender inequalities.

Pregnancy and Childbirth

Complications from pregnancy are the leading cause of death for young women ages 15 through 19 in low- and middle-income countries. Throughout the world, 200 million women wish to avoid or delay pregnancy, but they do not have access to modern methods of contraception.

Maternal health and the health of the child are closely related. A child whose mother dies has a risk of death that is three to ten times greater than the risk for a child whose mother is alive. Every year, more than 50 million women, including 60% of women in sub-Saharan Africa and 70% in South Asia, give birth at home without the help of a trained attendant, which endangers the health of both the mothers and their newborn.

The most common cause of maternal death is bleeding, which can cause death even for a healthy woman within two hours if it is not attended to. Timely and competent care is the key to saving the life of a woman who is hemorrhaging after giving birth. Sepsis and unsafe abortions are the second and third most frequent causes of maternal deaths worldwide.

Access to Birth Control

An estimated 150 million women worldwide do not have access to the birth control that they desire. As a result many women or girls have babies at young ages that they cannot care for, or they have illegal abortions, which often are fatal for the women.

Factors for barriers to birth control:

- lack of education about contraception,
- limited choices,
- high costs,
- limited supplies,
- distance to services,
- cultural, religious, or personal objections.

In many cultures and regions of the world, the right of a woman to choose when and how many children she will have is viewed as someone else's decision or right.

What Is the Global Gag Rule?

The U.S. Mexico City Policy, also known as the Global Gag Rule, banned all foreign nongovernmental organizations from receiving financial support from the United States if they did any of the following things:

- counseled clients about abortion,
- referred clients for abortion,
- lobbied their own governments to either make abortion legal or easier to obtain in their countries.

The Gag Rule denied funding to these organizations when they broke the rules of the U.S. policy, even when those actions were legal in the country, and even when they were paid for with other funds not from the U.S. government. This policy was funded under the Bush administration.

In 2009, President Obama repealed the Global Gag Rule through executive order, removing restrictions on which organizations are eligible for U.S. family planning assistance. He has also expressed support for comprehensive sex education within the United States.

In his 2009 budget blueprint, President Obama called for, "increasing investments in global health programs, including areas such as maternal and child health, family planning, and other core health programs."

Anemia

Anemia is a deficiency of red blood cells and/or hemoglobin that decreases the ability of the blood to transfer oxygen to the tissues in the body. Anemia is most prevalent among women, infants, and children because pregnancy and growth increase the body's demand for iron. The WHO estimates that 2 billion people in the world are anemic.

Approximately half of all cases of anemia are a result of dietary iron deficiency caused by an inadequate intake of and poor absorption of iron. Anemia also can be caused by infections, malaria, genetic disorders such as sickle cells, and blood loss during childbirth.

Interventions to decrease anemia among women include the following:

- iron supplements for women who are pregnant and adolescent girls,
- the reduction of malaria and hookworms, and
- efforts to ensure that a mother leaves adequate time between the births of children, as a mother who gives birth too soon after a previous birth can suffer severe anemia and can bleed to death.

Gender-Based Violence

Gender-based violence is a major public health and human rights concern in many societies throughout the world. Rape, domestic violence, child marriage, sex trafficking, and female genital mutilation are just a few of the abuses that women and girls are force to suffer. Wars are currently raging in many parts of the world, and about 90% of those injured or killed in these conflicts are civilians, 75% of whom are women and children. Millions of women caught up in the midst of wars are raped or forced to endure other types of violence, displaced from their own homes, lose loved ones, or are suddenly forced to become the sole provider for their families.

Violence against women is one of the four general causes of death in the world today, along with disease, hunger, and war, according to the head of a Swiss defense institute that recently published a study entitled "Women in an Insecure World." Swiss Ambassador Theodor Winkler, Director of the Geneva Center for the Democratic Control of Armed Forces, has stated that the number of women who die as a result of gender-related violence, deprivation, and discrimination is greater than the number of casualties in all the wars of the twentieth century combined.

Winkler went on to say that approximately 80 million of the 200 million missing females are the result of abortions of female fetuses in societies in which boys have a higher value than girls. The report notes that medical testing for **sex selection,** although it has been officially banned, has become "a booming business" in China, India, and South Korea, all of which now have significantly fewer girls than boys.

The World Health Organizations (WHO) World Report on Violence and Health notes that one of the most common forms of violence against women is domestic violence. This type of violence is frequently invisible because it happens behind closed doors in the privacy of homes, and many legal systems and cultural norms do not treat such violence as crimes, but rather as "private" family matters or a normal part of domestic life.

An **honor killing** is a murder of a woman who has been perceived as having brought dishonor to her family. Honor killings are typically committed by the victim's own relatives and/or community, and, unlike crimes of passion or rage-induced killings, they are usually planned in advance. **An honor suicide** occurs when a woman who is considered to be disgraced is ordered or pressured into killing herself. Hundreds, if not thousands, of women are murdered by their families every year for the sake of family "honor." This practice cuts across some cultures and religions. Honor killings occur in Bangladesh, Brazil, Ecuador, Egypt, India, Israel, Jordan, Pakistan, Morocco, Turkey, Uganda, Iran, and Iraq. It is estimated that every day in Pakistan, at least three women are victims of honor killings, and in India, more than 5,000 brides die annually because their dowries are considered to be insufficient.

Honor killings are performed for a wide variety of reasons. Marital infidelity, pre-marital sex, flirting, and even failing to serve a meal on time can all be perceived as bringing shame upon a family. Amnesty International even reported one case in which a husband murdered his wife based on a dream that she had betrayed him. In Turkey, a young woman's throat was cut in a public square because a love ballad had been dedicated to her on the radio.

Female Genital Mutilation

Female genital mutilation, often referred to as female circumcision, involves the partial or complete removal of the external female genitalia or other injuries to female genital organs for cultural, religious, or other non-medical reasons. Today, the number of girls and women who have undergone female genital mutilation is between 100 and 140 million. It is estimated that a further 2 million girls are at risk of having to undergo female genital mutilation.

Most girls and women who have undergone genital mutilation live in 28 African countries, although some live in Asia and, the Middle East. In addition, some immigrants from these countries and regions to Europe, Australia, Canada, and the United States also have undergone this procedure, which is usually performed by a traditional practitioner with instruments such as knives and other blades and without any type of anesthetic. The age at which female genital mutilation is performed varies from infants who are only a few days old, to female children and adolescents and, occasionally, to mature women. Refusal to undergo the procedure may jeopardize a woman's family relationships, her social life, and her ability to find a spouse.

Female genital mutilation is performed for the following reasons:

- to maintain chastity and virginity before marriage and fidelity during marriage:
- to increase male sexual pleasure;
- to have the females identify with their cultural heritage;
- because external female genitalia are considered dirty and unsightly; and
- because of the notion that women's bodies are inherently flawed and require correction.

Health Consequences of Female Genital Mutilation:

- severe pain,
- shock,
- hemorrhage,
- ulceration of the genital region and injury to adjacent tissue,
- infection that can cause death,

- cysts and abscesses,
- scar formation,
- damage to the urethra, resulting in urinary incontinence,
- pain during sexual intercourse and sexual dysfunction,
- difficulties with childbirth, and
- possible transmission of HIV when one instrument is used in multiple operations.

Genital mutilation can leave lasting marks on the lives and minds of women who have undergone it. In the long term, these women may suffer feelings of incompleteness, anxiety, and depression.

Ending Female Genital Mutilation

The Torture Convention defines **torture** as "any act by which severe pain or suffering, whether physical or mental, is intentionally inflicted on a person." An unauthorized invasion or alteration of a person's body represents a disregard for that person's fundamental right. Respect for women's dignity implies acceptance of their physical qualities, including the natural appearance of their genitalia and their normal sexual functions. A decision to alter those qualities should not be imposed upon a woman or girl for the purpose of reinforcing socially defined roles. Similarly, because female genital mutilation is an intervention into one of the most intimate aspects of a woman's life, her sexuality, the practice of genital mutilation violates her rights to privacy. It is also a form of violence against women, because in some cases it is performed despite a woman's protests or before she has attained the age of consent, which varies among different countries.

Violence against women is being addressed at the international level as a human rights issue. UNICEF and the United Nations Development Fund for Women have programs in place that address the issue. However, much work needs to be done at local levels. Increased public awareness and greater education about female genital mutilation is definitely needed.

Human Trafficking

Human trafficking for the purpose of sexual exploitation has become a part of international organized crime and generates high profits with low risks for traffickers. The United Nations estimates that 4 million people are bought and sold each year, resulting in $7 billion in profits to criminal organizations. Many countries have no laws or very weak ones against human trafficking, thus making it less risky and more profitable to criminals than trafficking in drugs or weapons. Trafficking networks may buy, abduct, or lure girls and women with promises of a better life in another country, only to transport them to places where they essentially work as slaves in forced prostitution, sweatshop labor, and in private homes as servants.

Several factors lead women to look for potential work in other countries. Globalization has resulted in an increase in poverty among females, forcing greater numbers of women in various countries to emigrate in search of work. Seeking job opportunities abroad, some women turn to newspaper ads, acquaintances, marriage agencies, labor recruiters, and modeling agencies, which many times intentionally mislead these women and trick them into accepting positions as nannies, maids, dancers, factory workers, and hostesses. These positions often are fake; the women are transported to another country, where they do not speak the language, their passports have been taken, and they end up as slaves.

Trafficking in women has been increasing in Eastern Europe, particularly Ukraine, and in Africa, Southeast Asia, from which countries the women are transported to North America. The majority of child trafficking occurs in Asia, although it is a global problem. In Thailand, up to one-third of prostitutes are children and adolescents under the age of 18. Nepal's extreme poverty and its economic and political relationship with India have facilitated the trafficking of Nepali women and girls to brothels in India.

Debt bondage is a situation in which debtors pledge their personal services against a debt that they owe, but the person to whom they owe the debt fails to deduct the value of their services from the debt, or does not limit and define the length and nature of those services. For example, if a mother with no money has a child who is ill and in need of medicine, she might get a loan from one of those debtors and will then be forced to pay off the debt by becoming a slave. Unfortunately, the debtors ensure that the debts are never paid off.

Ending Human Trafficking

Federal trafficking legislation has only been in place in the United States since 2000. It provides for strict penalties for human traffickers and gives victims a variety of benefits, including a special temporary visa for three years. A victim can receive medical counseling, psychological counseling, and emergency shelter. However, to receive these benefits, a victim must testify against her traffickers—something that most girls and women, out of fear of retaliation, will not do. Although the 2000 laws are a start, more pressure must be placed on the federal government to protect and aid the victims of human trafficking without penalties.

Rape Used as a Weapon of War in Darfur

The United Nations (UN) Humanitarian Coordinator has called the genocide in Darfur the worst humanitarian crisis of the twenty-first century. The crisis has led to the displacement of at least 1.2 million people and the deaths of 400,000. Not since the Rwandan genocide of 1994 has the world seen such a calculated campaign of mass slaughter, rape, displacement, and starvation. The humanitarian crisis of Darfur was directly caused by war crimes and crimes against humanity, for which the Sudanese government is responsible. Illegal attacks on civilians in northern, western, and southern states in Darfur by a government-sponsored militia commonly referred to as "Janjaweed" (armed men on horses) or "Arab militia," and by the government army. In these attacks, men are killed, women are raped, and villagers are forcibly displaced from their homes, which are set on fire. Their crops and cattle, their main means of subsistence, are also burned. Many people who have been displaced live in temporary camps and have little access to health care. Overcrowding, food shortages and outbreaks or disease are common conditions in these camps.

Human rights violations that have specifically targeted women and girls in Darfur include abductions, sexual slavery, torture, and forced displacement.

The testimonies collected by Amnesty International indicate that rape and other forms of sexual violence are being used as weapons of war in Darfur to humiliate, punish, control, cause fear, and displace women and their families. Even pregnant women have not been spared. Amnesty International has reported cases in which the Janjaweed killed women precisely because they were pregnant.

Every day, women are sent outside the camps to seek firewood and water, despite the constant risk of rape at the hands of the Janjaweed. If men were to venture out of the camps, they would risk castration and murder. Faced with such an inhumane choice, families usually decide that rape is the lesser evil.

In other cases, the Janjaweed have tortured women to force them to disclose the locations where their husbands are hiding. Forms of torture reportedly have included putting the face of a woman between two wooden sticks and squeezing hard, and pulling out the nails of their fingers and toes. Some women have also reported that the Janjaweed broke the the legs of rape victims to prevent them from escaping.

Rape has many consequences, some of which have immediate effects and some of which have long-term effects on women, in addition to the actual physical violation of the rape itself. Rape in itself is a heinous violation of human rights, but its victims are likely to suffer further because of the shame and stigma associated with it. Violence, sexual and otherwise, can cause serious damage to women's reproductive systems. The physical and psychological violence of rape on women who are already pregnant can lead to miscarriages and spontaneous abortions. In such cases, women are sometimes rejected even by their husbands, as they are not seen as fulfilling their roles as reproducers. For women who have undergone female genital mutilation, the risk of injuries during rape increases, and consequently so does the risk of women contracting HIV/AIDS or other sexually transmitted diseases. At the present time, there are very few medical facilities that can provide adequate medical care for women who are victims of violent rapes.

In Darfur, children are considered to be mainly the responsibility of women; hence, violence against children has considerably traumatized women. Children are killed and abducted, reportedly in large numbers. Children also suffer when their mothers or fathers are killed in the conflict and when they are separated from their families.

Children are particularly at risk of malnutrition, diarrhea, malaria, and other ailments. An estimated 80% of the displaced children under 5 years of age are suffering from severe malnutrition, and 70% of the deaths in the camps are of children under age 5.

How to stop the genocide:

If you understand that genocide is occurring right now, it is also your responsibility as a human to look for ways to stop the genocide. These people need our help.

- Millions of investors are unaware that their savings are invested in companies that help fund genocide in Darfur. Divest for Darfur is a national campaign to encourage investment firms, especially J.P. Morgan, Franklin Templeton, Fidelity Investments, Capital Group (American Funds), and Vanguard to withdraw investments from companies that help fund genocide in Darfur. Go to savedarfur.org/divest for more information.
- Educate friends, neighbors, and others in your community about the genocide that is occurring.
- Call, write to, or e-mail your concerns about this issue to your representative in Congress.
- For further information, go to www.savedarfur.org and www.standnow.org.

Ending Violence against Women through Education and Empowerment

Much violence is tied into the economic slavery of women. Millions of women in the world are plagued by not having enough money to live on, which keeps them imprisoned in violent relationships. Jobs that provide living wages need to be created for women to help them become independent. Another means of help is to assist women with planning their families and futures. Family planning services allow women to decide if, when, and how often they wish to have children.

Family planning funding has decreased by about 40% in real terms since 1995. At the same time, the adolescent population has grown and is expected to continue to do so over the next two decades. Family planning programs reduce maternal and newborn mortality, unintended pregnancies, and incidences of unsafe abortions.

> ***"The problems we face today, violent conflicts, destruction of nature, poverty, hunger and so on, are human-created pro6lems which can be resolved through human effort, understanding and the development of a sense of brotherhood and sisterhood. We need to cultivate a universal responsibility for one another and the planet we share."***
>
> ***—the Dalai Lama***

Decreasing the devastating impact of infectious diseases can prevent deaths and improve the quality of lives throughout the world. Proven and cost-effective medicines, vaccines, and other products and methods do exist to prevent and treat illnesses.

Some of the best health-care solutions are as simple and inexpensive as teaching mothers to keep their newborns clean and warm; advising people at risk of heart disease to eat a low-fat diet; and educating people about the importance of using condoms to avoid being infected with HIV. Many health-care interventions—such as curbing tobacco use and improving nutrition—target several health problems at once.

The most cost-effective interventions include the following:

- **Provide bed nets** treated with insecticide ($4.80 per bed net). Malaria is transmitted by mosquitoes almost exclusively at night. Bed nets have been proven to control the spread of the disease in endemic regions.
- **Provide water purification systems** ($0.04 per sachet). More than 1 billion people in the world do not have access to safe drinking water. Simple household water treatments can stop the spread of deadly water-borne diseases such as cholera. PUR packets from Procter and Gamble are very effective in purifying drinking water in developing countries.

- **Increase condom availability** ($1 or less per condom). The best way to stop the spread of HIV and STDs is still prevention. Behavioral changes and condom use can decrease the global pandemic of HIV/AIDS.
- **Vaccinate poor children against measles** ($0.13 per dose). The measles vaccine is safe, inexpensive, and almost 100% effective. Yet in many developing countries, children still do not have access to these vaccines, and, as a result, 500,000 to 700,000 children die each year from this preventable disease, while many others suffer lifelong disabilities, including blindness, deafness, and brain damage.
- **Tax tobacco products** to increase their price and thus motivate people to quit smoking, which will reduce the prevalence of cardiovascular disease, cancer, and respiratory diseases. Tobacco is the second major cause of death in the world—killing one in 10 adults worldwide, or about 5 million people each year.
- **Attack the spread of HIV** by promoting condom use among populations at high risk; treating other sexually transmitted diseases; providing antiretroviral medications, especially for pregnant women; and offering voluntary HIV/AIDS counseling and testing.
- **Make sure that children and pregnant women receive essential nutrients**, including vitamin A, iron, and iodine to prevent maternal anemia, infant deaths, and other long-term health problems.
- **Treat TB patients** with antibiotics and short-term chemotherapy.
- **Promote the use of aspirin** in adults and behavioral changes such as a healthful diet and exercise to treat and prevent heart attack and stroke.

Conclusion

It's tough to be a young person today and to look at the problems of the world without completely losing hope. What I have found in my life to help me get through those times is to participate. Anything that you can do to get involved will help you feel more connected to the world. It is precisely during these trying times that the United States needs its best and brightest young people, from all walks of life, to step forward and commit to public service. Times like these call for people to stand up and get to work. To break barriers and to drive change, roll up your sleeves instead of throwing up your hands. Because of globalization, our world is so small that you cannot ignore the genocide in Darfur, or the fact that one out of every eight American is living in poverty, with millions more struggling just to get by. You cannot turn away as pandemic diseases torment the people of entire continents. And you can't look aside as citizens are denied their most basic human rights, such as safe food, water, and access to health care.

When it comes to public health, lives are often saved, or dramatically improved, by the things that cost the least. Simple undertakings—such as washing hands, using a seatbelt, quitting smoking, eating more fruits and vegetables and less fat and sugar—have little or no cost to an individual. However, collectively, such actions can make a huge difference in public health.

References

Abreu A. G., Noguer I., & Cowgill K., "HIV/AIDS in Latin American Countries," *The World Bank http://go.worldbank.org/KIC4QIMK20*

A Joint Assessment of HIV/AIDS Prevention, Treatment and Care in China, State Council HIV/AIDS Working Committee Office and UN Theme Group on HIV/AIDS in China, 2003. http://www.unaids.org.cn/uploadfiles/20080725151739.pdf

Bryce, J., Boschi-Pinto, C., Shibuya, K., & Black, R.E., (WHO Child Health Epidemiology Reference Group: "WHO estimates the causes of death in children," *Lancet* 365(9465) (2005): 1147–1152.

BBC News, "Cuba to help Caribbean fight AIDS," Jul;y 16, 2004.

Bogart, L. M., & Thorburn, S., "Are HIV/AIDS conspiracy beliefs a barrier to HIV prevention among African Americans?" *Journal of Acquired Immune Deficiency Syndromes,* 38(2) (2005): 213–218.

Bronfman, M.N., et al. (2002), "Mobile populations and IIIV/AIDS in Central America and Mexico: research for action," *AIDS:* vol. 16 Supplement 3, December 2002, S42–S49.

Campbell, O.M.R., & W.J. Graham. "Strategies for reducing maternal mortality: getting on with what works," *Lancet* 368 (2006): 2121–2122.

Centers for Disease Control and Prevention, *HIV/AIDS Surveillance Report* 7 (2). (Atlanta: U.S. Department of Health and Human Services, Centers for Disease Control and Prevention, 1995), http://www.cdc.gov/hiv/stats/hasrlink.htm.

Centers for Disease Control and Prevention, *HIV/AIDS Among African Americans Fact Sheet* (Atlanta: U.S. Department of Health and Human Services, Centers for Disease Control and Prevention, 2005) http://Jwww.cdc.gov/hiv/.

Centers for Disease Control and Prevention, HIV/AIDS Surveillance Report, 15 (Atlanta: U.S. Department of Health and Human Services, Centers for Disease Control and Prevention, 2003), http://www.cdc.gov/hiv/stats/.

Centers for Disease Control and Prevention, *HIV/AIDS among Youth Fact Sheet* (Atlanta: U.S. Department of Health and Human Services, Centers for Disease Control and Prevention, 2005), http://www.cdc.gov/hiv/pubs/facts/youth.htm.

Centers for Disease Control and Prevention, *HIV/AIDS Among Women Fact Sheet* (Atlanta: U.S. Department of Health and Human Services, Centers for Disease Control and Prevention, 2004), http://www.cdc.gov/hiv/pubs/facts/women.htm.

Centers for Disease Control and Prevention, *HIV/AIDS Among Men Who Have Sex with Men Fact Sheet.* (Atlanta: U.S. Department of Health and Human Services, Centers for Disease Control and Prevention, 2005).

Centers for Disease Control and Prevention, *HIV/AJDS Surveillance Report, 2005,* vol. 17. (Atlanta: U.S. Department of Health and Human Services, CDC, 2006), 1–46.

Channel 4, UK, *Dying for Drugs,* April 27, 2003.

Cohen, J., "The overlooked epidemic," *Science* vol. 313 Issue 5786, July 28, 2006.

Cohen, J., "Mexico: Prevention programs target migrants," *Science* vol. 313 Issue 5786, July 28, 2006.

Cohen, J., "Haiti: Making headway under hellacious circumstances," *Science* vol. 313 Issue 5786, July28, 2006.

Colgan, Ann-Louise, "Hazardous to health: The World Bank and IMF in Africa," *Africa Action,* April 18, 2002.

DeParle,J. "Talk of government being out to get blacks falls on more attentive ears," *The New York Times,* Oct. 29, 1990.

Disease Control Priorities Project, "Best buys and priorities for action in developing countries," *Investing in Global Health,* April 2006.

Fawthrop, T,:Cuba: Is it a model in HIV/AIDS battle?" London Panes, 2003).

Fink, S., "Cuba's energetic AIDS doctor," *American Journal of Public Health,* 93(5) (2003): 712–716.

Frasca, T.,, "AIDS in Latin America," (Hampshire: Paigrave/Macmillan,2005) 144.

Goldstein, Matthew A, "The biological roots of heat-of-passion crimes and honor killings," *Politics and the Life Sciences,* vol. 21, no 2, September 2002, 28–37.

Ghosh, T.K., "AIDS: A serious challenge to public health," *Journal of the Indian Medical Association,* 84(1) (1986): 29–30.

Hacker, M., Malta, M., Enriquez, M., et al., "Human immunodeficiency virus, AIDS, and drug consumption in South America and the Carribean: Epidenilological evidence and initiatives to curb the epidemic," *Rev Panam Salud Publica,*18(4/5) (2005): 303–313.

Henry J. Kaiser Foundation, *Global Health Facts, Menlo Park:* 2009. http://www.KaiserEDU.org");

Human Rights Watch, "Jordan Parliament Supports Impunity for Honor Killing," Press Release, Washington. D.C.: January 2000.

Jamison, D. T., J. G. Breman, A. R. Measham, G. Alleyne, M. Claeson, D. B. Evans, P. Jha, A. Mills, & P. Musgrove, *Disease Control Priorities in Developing Countries* (2nd ed.) (New York: Oxford University Press, 2006).

Jamison, D. T., J. G. Breman, A. R. Measham, G. Alleyne, M. Claeson, D. B. Evans, P. Jha, A. Mills, & P. Musgrove, *Priorities in Health.* (Washington, D.C.: World Bank, 2006).

Jarosewich, Irene, "Reports on trafficking of women in Europe: Most who seek rescue are from Ukraine," *The Ukrainian Weekly,* no. 32, vol. LXVI, August 9, 1998, at http://www.ukrweekly.com/Archive/1998/329802.shtnil.

Jyothi Kanics, "Trafficking in Women," *Global Survival Network*, eds. Tom Barry (LRC) and Martha Honey (IPS) *In Focus* 3(30) (October 1998), at http://www.foreignpolicyinfocus.or Jbriefs/vol3/v3n30wom.html.

Kanics, Jyothi, "Foreign Policy in Focus: Trafficking in Women," *Global Survival Network* vol. 3, no. 30, October 1998;

Kakar, D.N., and Kakar, S.N., "Combating AIDS in the 21st century issues and challenges," (New York: Sterling Publishers Private Limited, 2001) 31.

Lawn, J.E., Cousens, S,, Darmstadt, G.L., Bhutta, Z., Martines, J., Paul, V,, et al, "1 year after The Lancet Neonatal Survival Series—was the call for action heard?" *Lancet*;367 (2006):1541–1547.

Lawn, J.E., Cousens, S., & Zupan, J., "4 million neonatal deaths: When? where? why?" *Lancet*;365 (2005): 891–900.

Lopez, A. D., C. D. Mathers, M. Ezzati, D. T. Jamison, & C. J. L. Murray, *Global Burden of Disease and Risk Factors* (New York: Oxford University Press, 2006).

National Alliance of State and Territorial AIDS Directors, *HIV/AIDS: African American Perspectives and Recommendations for State and Local AIDS Directors and Health Departments,* 2001.

New York Times, "How to avoid honor killing in Turkey? Honor Suicide, July 16, 2006.

Pope, Victoria, "Trafficking in women: Procuring Russians for sex abroad—even in America." *US News and World Report*, April 7, 1997, at, http://www.usnews.cornIusnews/issue/970407/7ring.htm.

Ronsmans, Carine, &Wendy J. Graham, "Maternal mortality: Who, when, where and why." The Lancet 368 (2006): 1189–1199.

Robert E. Black, Saul S. Morris, & Jennifer Bryce, "Where and why are 10 million children dying every year?" *The Lancet*, vol. 361, no. 9376, June 28, 2003.

Specter, Michael, "Contraband women—A special report: Traffickers" new cargo: Naive slavic women," *The New York Times.* January 11, 1998.

The Hemy J. Kaiser Family Foundation and the National Alliance of State and Territorial AIDS Directors, *National ADAP Monitoring Project* (Annual Report), 2005., http://www.kff.org/hivaids/7288.cfm.

The Kaiser Family Foundation, *Kaiser Family Foundation Survey of Americans on HIV/A1DS: Part Three—Experiences and Opinions by Race/Ethnicity and Ag*, August, 2004,. http://www.kff.org/hivaids/upload/44743_l.pdf.

The Kaiser Family Foundation, *African Americans and HIV/AIDS* (HIV/AIDS Policy Fact Sheet), Feb. 2005,. http://www.kff.org/hivaidsl.

The Kaiser Family Foundation, *The Uninsured: A Primer - Key Facts About Americans Without Health Insurance,* Nov. 2004, http://www.kff.org/uninsured/72l6.cfm?\.

The Lancet, "Spreading the word about HIV/AIDS in India," vol. 361, May 3, 2003.

The Rutherford Institute 4/10/06) http:/Jwww.rutherford.orglarticles_db/commentary.asp?record_id=397

UNAIDS/WHO 2006 AIDS epidemic update http://www.unaids.org/en/KnowledgeCentre/HIVData/EpiUpdate/EpiUpdArchive/2006/default.asp

UNAIDS, *A Study of the Pan Caribbean Partnership against HIV/AIDS (PANCAP) Common Goals, Shared Responses,*. December, 2004., http://data.unaids.org/publications/IRC-pub06/jc1089-pancap_en.pdf

UNAIDS, *UNAIDS at Country Level: Progress Report 2004* http://data.unaids.org/pub/Report/2006/2006_country_progress_report_burundi_en.pdf

UNICEF,*State of the World's Children,* 2005–2007., http://www.unicef.org/eapro/Human_Development_in_Crisis.pdf.

UNICEF, "Statistics: Under 5 Mortality Rate," at http://www.childinfo.org/areas/childmortality/u5data.php.

UNESCO, *EFA Global Monitoring Report.* (Paris: UNESCO, 2007).

U.S. Department of Justice, *Bureau of Justice Statistics Bulletin: Prison and Jail Inmates at Midyear 2004.* (Washington, D.C.: U.S. Department of Justice, 2005), at http://www.ojp.usdoj.gov/bjs/.

U.S. Department of Health and Human Services, "China urges needle exchanges, free condoms in new AIDS strategy", Associated Press, 7 June 2005

U.S. Department of Justice, (2004, December), Bureau of Justice Statistics Bulletin: HIV in Prisons and Jails, 2002. http://www.ojp.usdoj .gov/bjs/pub/pdf7hivpj02 .pdf

Wongsrichanalai C, Barcus MJ, Muth S, Sutamihardja A, Wernsdorfer WH. 2007. A review of malaria diagnostic tools: microscopy and rapid diagnostic test (RDT). *Am J Trop Med Hyg* 77(Suppl 6):119–27.

World Bank (2000) "Thailand's Response to AIDS: Building on Success, Confronting the Future", Thailand social Monitor V, p.10–il

World Development Index 2002, The World Bank

World Health Organization Fact sheet No 104, March 2007; http://www.who.org

World Health Organization, *Economic costs of malgfr, November 27, 2005*

World Health Organization (17 April 2007), 'Towards Universal Access: Scaling up priority HIV/AIDS interventions in the health sector'

WHO. 2005. Make every mother and child count. Geneva: WHO.

WHO. 2005. Facts and figures form the World Health Report 2005. Geneva: WHO.

Women's Human Rights Resources at http ://www.law-lib.utoronto .caiDianai

Zipperer M. (July 2005), 'HIV/AIDS Prevention and Control: the Cuban Response', The Lancet Infectious Diseases, Volume 5, Issue 7